Nonverbal Communication with Patients:

Back to the Human Touch

Nonverbal Communication with Patients:

Back to the Human Touch

Marion Nesbitt Blondis, R.N., M.A.
Professor of Nursing, Emeritus
College of the Desert
Palm Desert, California

Barbara E. Jackson, B.A.
Director, Institute of Medical Studies
Los Angeles, California

A Wiley Medical Publication
John Wiley & Sons
New York • London • Sydney • Toronto

Library of Congress Cataloging in Publication Data:

Blondis, Marion N
    Nonverbal communication with patients.

    (A Wiley medical publication)
    Bibliography: p.
    Includes index.
    1. Nurse and patient. 2. Nonverbal
communication (psychology) 3. Communication in
nursing. I. Jackson, Barbara E., joint author.
II. Title. [DNLM: 1. Nonverbal communication—
Nursing texts. 2. Nurse-patient relations.
WY S7 B654n]
RT86.B55   610.73'069   76-30732
ISBN 0-471-01753-1

Printed in the United States of America

10 9 8 7 6 5 4 3 2

Foreword

All too often a public exposed to television and movie portrayals of hospital scenes depicting nurses in starched white uniforms, functioning amidst a myriad of tubes, electronic monitors, push-button communicators, and complicated scanners, stereotypes them as machine-oriented, cold practitioners. Nurses, themselves, attempting to perform skillfully their role with the expertise these technologic innovations demand, may lose sight of their prime desire to administer total care encompassing the emotional needs of patients and concurrently satisfy personal needs for accomplishment. Thus, *Nonverbal Communication with Patients: Back to the Human Touch* is a refreshingly warm, humanistic answer to the dilemma nurses encounter in struggling with this dichotomy between mechanistic efficiency and tender caring.

In this book the importance of nonverbal communication is thoroughly explored in chapters on the observational skills pertinent to data gathering to determine covert problems in assessing the nursing diagnosis. Based on the research of Darwin, of Birdwhistle, and of Hall, the concept of nonverbal communication is expanded beyond kinetics—physical movements or expressions—to include proxemics—spatial concepts that have only recently entered the therapeutic milieu.

The mutuality of interaction and the nuances of the nurse's expressions as an emission of feelings which console or increase anxiety are skillfully explained. The difficulties that nurses encounter in their interaction with patients, not the least of which are their own humanness and consequent imperfections, are also realistically handled. The first chapter describes the need for properly interpreting the cardiac patient's fears by eye contact, downcast lips, tremorous fingers. In subsequent chapters the authors explicitly consider pertinent problems encountered throughout the life cycle. Topics such as communication in medical nursing, pediatric nursing, mothering, geriatric nursing, death and dying, and times of crisis are thoroughly discussed, with realistic situations presented as a basis for practical resolutions. Such "touchy" subjects as sexual manifestations of the patient which may confuse and embarrass the nurse are treated in detail. Valid authorities provide the philosophic basis for the pediatric content especially, which leans heavily on the works of Escalona, Spitz, and Erikson.

The lucidity of the text, while displaying depth and scholarliness, will appeal to readers with a wide range of backgrounds. The realistic, practical, and imaginative aids suggested by the authors in problem situations can be a stimulus for emulation or a catalyst to more innovative practitioners intent on "doing their own thing" in striving to achieve their goals within the scope of the independent nursing functions.

A valuable supplement to a basic nursing text for the beginning student, this admirable work will continue to be useful throughout the nurse's professional career. Truly the book fulfills a long-felt need. It is hoped, too, that it may serve to enhance the public image of the nurse.

SYLVIA LASSER
Associate Professor of Nursing
Nassau Community College
Garden City, New York

Preface

My years of instructing young nurses taught me that the brightest or the most academically gifted students did not always develop into the best nurses. Frequently, there was an ingredient missing—human understanding, feeling for the patient's emotional needs. I became engrossed in the question of how best to convey to my students that there is something more to bedside nursing than simply following hospital procedures. I tried to teach them that it is equally important to understand the procedures of human relationships. Because of this interest, I did my graduate work in human behavior. I determined that communication was the crux, but that communication consisted of more than the spoken word. Words are like the lines of a painting; nonverbal action fills out the picture with color and shade. I began to focus on nonverbal communication and ran experimental testing with my students. I soon learned that nonverbal communication is teachable. In a conversation one spring morning with Anne Roe, Wiley author, I asked what her feelings were on the possibility of a book on nonverbal communication for nurses. Her enthusiastic response started me on the journey toward publication. Writing was a new world to me, so I enlisted the help of my very capable coauthor, Barbara Jackson; without her efforts the ideas would not have found words.

MARION NESBITT BLONDIS, R.N.

Palm Springs, California
August 1976

ix

Acknowledgments

Thanks to Marian Katz, R.N., M.A., Betty Jo Marshall, R.N., M.V.E., Kathleen Chapin, R.N., B.S., Eleanor Johnson, R.N., Myrtle Jackson, R.N., and Joy Ufema, R.N., who served as resource people. Thanks also to Earl Shepherd, Former Editor, Wiley; and to Jeanne.

Special thanks to Mary Dispenza, Principal, St. Mary's Elementary School, Aberdeen, Washington, for the creativity of her art form which is found in this book; and to Margaret Lockhart, R.N., who gave so willingly of her time. Her typing and support have made this book possible. Special thanks also to Robert.

Our gratitude to Anne K. Roe, who started us on this journey toward publication.

M.N.B. and B.E.J.

Contents

Nonverbal Communication with Patients:

Back to the Human Touch

1

What Is Nonverbal Communication?

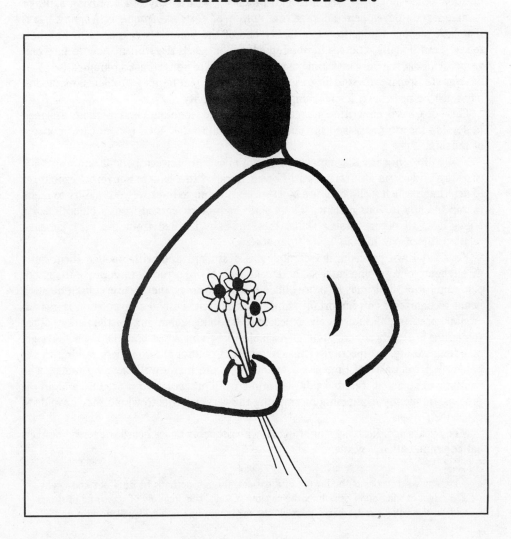

The face of nursing has changed drastically over the past few decades. At the turn of the century, many now controllable diseases were fatal. The nurse could only stand by helplessly and make the dying patient's last hours as comfortable as possible. She could care for the patient. Indeed, the very word "nurse" was defined as "someone trained to care for the sick." In our own century, many once-pressing medical riddles have been solved through research and technology. New cures and new life support systems call for new procedures, and nurses are required to master those procedures. Therefore, the emphasis in nursing has gradually shifted from the caring role to one of excellence in nursing skills, techniques, and procedures.

The procedures nurses perform must not take precedence over the *very human* beings for whom those activities are performed. When the patient is approached humanistically, significant therapeutic progress can be made. Nonverbal communication, intelligently understood, can be a most effective tool toward that goal. The nursing role involves more than good procedures and technical skills; there is a growing awareness that we, in nursing, must develop a sensitivity to the patient's emotional needs. Communication skills should be identified and practiced, just as any other nursing skills or techniques are developed. Thora Kron, author of *Communication in Nursing,*[1] says that lack of communication is probably one of the greatest weaknesses in hospitals today. Traditionally, courses in nursing education teach the student how to interpret verbal symbols, but very little time, if any, is devoted to nonverbal communication. Yet, if we are to prepare the student to solve today's very real nursing problems, methodology must be developed for teaching skills in sensitivity.

This book has been written in an attempt to define techniques and methods designed to develop the awareness and the sensitivity so vital to the "total patient care" concept of nursing.

You will soon learn that nonverbal communication between patient and nurse is a two-way bridge. As a nurse, you will be encouraged to evaluate nonverbal exchanges to determine which techniques are most successful and to improve your ability to relate therapeutically to your patients. These skills cannot be learned from a blueprint or a book. Like all other nursing skills, they must be learned from the very personal relationship of one human being to another.

You will learn procedural techniques as a student and will practice them daily throughout your nursing career. There is no lack of opportunity to improve them, but communication skills may be more difficult. In some areas, therapeutic communication is not recognized as an important clinical component. Patient conversation is considered unnecessary, and nurses are expected to be doing something for the patient. That something is usually concrete and identifiable, like giving a bed-bath, taking a vital sign, or administering an injection. This same school of thought considers talking to the patient a great waste of time. As a result, there are many well-meaning nurses who continue to go about their busy days bustling from procedure to procedure and, in the process, frequently frightening or angering the very patients to whom they have dedicated their lives.

Many years ago, Florence Nightingale, who probably never heard the term "nonverbal communication," wrote:

"A nurse who rustles is the horror of a patient, though perhaps he does not know why. The fidget of silk and of crinoline, the rattling of keys, the creaking of stays and of shoes, will do the patient more harm than all the medicines in the world will do him good."

Florence Nightingale may not have known the term "nonverbal communication", but she did understand the human heart and the behaviors that speak silently to it.

When you walk briskly and frowning into a patient's room, stick a cold thermometer in his mouth, and take his wrist roughly for a pulse, you have told that patient everything he needs to know about your feelings toward him. There is no nursing procedure that is not accompanied by communication—a word or an unspoken message. The patient's understanding of that message does influence the outcome of the procedure.

So it is not a question of whether or not you should use nonverbal communication. You already do! It is an intricate part of your daily life. You receive nonverbal messages (cues) when you respond to the warmth of a hug, a child's smile, or the tears of someone you love. No words are necessary. In turn, you send nonverbal messages to others by your frown, smile, or outstretched hand. All human beings respond to the unspoken feelings of warmth, acceptance, and love. The decision, therefore, is whether or not you will use this inborn ability to communicate nonverbally as a therapeutic tool in your nursing career.

NONVERBAL COMMUNICATION DEFINED _____

To use nonverbal communication effectively, you must first define it; that is not always easy, since it is subject to a variety of interpretations. Ray Birdwhistell, a pioneer in nonverbal research, is reported to have said that studying nonverbal communication is like studying noncardiac physiology. It is a good analogy, clearly illustrating the point. It is not easy to separate human interactions, making a diagnosis that concerns only nonverbal behavior and another that concerns only verbal behavior.

Communication is basically a system for sending and receiving messages. We send and receive thoughts and feelings. We can transmit these through verbal symbols—our spoken words. We say: "I have an idea, listen to me. . . . I'm sad, cold, hungry, tired." We also transmit when we laugh, frown, or cry. Our actions—our nonverbal cues— are being transmitted as clearly as our spoken words and are understood as readily.

Vocal symbols are not the only means we use to communicate. Facial expression, posture, body movements, tone, and appearance are all dimensions of nonverbal communication. They are also dimensions of verbal communication because they support, emphasize, or contradict what we are saying. Some vocal sounds such as sighs, whimpers, groans, moans, and screams are not really verbal symbols; while they are vocal in nature, they really belong more to the realm of nonverbal communication. This brings us back to Birdwhistell's point that there is no true dichotomy between verbal and nonverbal behavior; a study of one will include many elements of the other. F. E. X. Dance[2] takes the question a step further by claiming that nonverbal vocal sounds become verbal when they are heard and interpreted by someone. According to his theory, a scream is vocal sound, but it becomes verbal when a passerby hears it and interprets it as a cry for help. For the purposes of this book, we will examine the interaction between nonverbal and verbal communication, as well as the behaviors that are more exclusively nonverbal.

This would be a good time to explain some of the terms used in nonverbal communication. Knowledge of these terms will help you recognize the specific behaviors and their general categories.

Body Motion or Kinetic Behavior

Body motion (kinetic behavior) includes gestures, movements of the body, hands, head, feet, facial expression, eye behavior, and posture. There are different types of kinetic cues, just as there are different kinds of verbal symbols. Some body cues are specific; others are general. Some communicate, while others provide information about how we are feeling or about our personalities. Until recently, the field of kinetic behavior was relatively uncharted. In 1969, Paul Ekman and Wallace Friesen developed a system for classifying these behavioral acts and divided them into the following categories:

Emblems.   Nonverbal acts that have a direct verbal translation or verbal definition are referred to as emblems. Sign language used by the deaf is an example of emblems. A wave to a friend too distant to hear a spoken greeting is another. These gestures translate nonverbally and clearly.

Illustrators.   These are totally nonverbal acts that accompany speech. They display and illustrate what is said verbally and are generally intentional. When you smile while telling someone that you are happy, the smile is the illustrator. It gives emphasis to your words.

Affect displays.   Facial expressions that display emotional states are referred to as affect displays. The smile used in the above definition was also an affect display. These expressions can emphasize, contradict, or even be unrelated to the spoken word. They can be intentional or unintentional.

Regulators.   Nonverbal actions that regulate flow in a conversation are called regulators. They tell the speaker to continue, to stop, that we are for him, are in disagreement, and so on. Regulators consist mainly of head nods, facial expressions, and eye movements.

Adaptors.   Most difficult to define are the adaptors, because they involve so much speculation. They are thought to develop in childhood as an adaptive effort to satisfy needs and to reveal personal orientations or characteristics. Many restless hand, foot, and leg motions fall into this category. We are usually unaware of our own adaptor activity.

Physical characteristics.   We can include in this category such things as body shape, height, weight, hair color, skin tone, body odors, and appearance. These are constitutional factors and remain relatively unchanged during the period of an interaction.

Touching behavior.   Touching is a separate and very important dimension of nonverbal behavior. It relates to actual physical contact with others. Subcategories would include stroking, hitting, greetings, farewells, holding, guiding another's movements, and other specific physical encounters.

In addition to the Ekman–Friesen classification, we should include two important areas for definition.

Paralanguage

Paralanguage deals with how something is said, rather than what is said. A whole range of nonverbal cues are involved, such as voice quality, pitch, tone, and tempo— and vocal characteristics, including coughing, whining, clearing of the throat, and so on.

The Concept of Territoriality

The term "territoriality" has been used in the study of animal behavior for many years. Most behavioral scientists agree that territoriality exists in human beings. Under this heading, we would deal with spatial relationships, the belongings of man—including the space around him, the manipulation of objects, territorial instincts, and environmental factors.

Recognizing Nonverbal Terminology

A quick examination of this list provides a brief introduction to the special terminology of nonverbal communication. The importance of nonverbal behaviors to the nursing environment cannot be covered in an encyclopedic definition of the categories. In nursing, we speak of caring for the patient. What do we really mean? A great deal of contemporary nursing literature postulates that empathy, compassion, and love are necessary and vital components of a meaningful and therapeutic nurse–patient relationship. The nurse should overtly project an attitude of understanding and unequivocal acceptance in order to nurse significantly and insightfully, e.g., she should actively demonstrate that she cares. This creates a problem in nursing because caring cannot be measured in the same terms as other nursing functions. The nurse knows that her message of caring is effective only when she observes the patient's response. Caring is communicated, verbally or nonverbally. Most nurses are aware of their verbal behavior (spoken words) with patients, but many nurses are apt to be unaware of their nonverbal behavior. Nonverbal communication is two-way communication. It communicates the nurse's feelings and intent to the patient and the patient's feelings and intent to the nurse. Nonverbal communication, therefore, is an important component of nursing because it conveys data about the patient to the nurse observer, and caring from nurse practitioner to patient.

The Nursing Care Situation

Understanding nonverbal communication is crucial to accurate nursing observation. Ida Jean Orlando in her text *The Dynamic Nurse–Patient Relationship*[3] defines four practices that are essential to basic nursing: (1) observations, (2) reporting, (3) recording, and (4) actions.

Observations are either direct or indirect. Indirect knowledge is derived from a source other than personal observation such as charts, nursing notes, and comments from physicians and other medical service personnel. Direct knowledge is defined as personal observation—any perception, thought, or feeling that the nurse has from her own experience of the patient's behavior.

All nursing procedures are designed to benefit the patient but, if they do not suit him because at that moment he requires something different, the procedure loses its desired effect. Too much medication when the patient does not need it will not benefit him any more than too little medication will when he does need it. The patient's needs change, and it is through nursing observation that those changes are met. Understanding nonverbal communication is crucial to the effectiveness of the nurse as an observer. With this relevance in mind, some additional exploration of nonverbal behaviors in the hospital environment is needed.

Touch (Tactile Communication)

In nursing, touch may be the most important of all nonverbal behaviors.

Patients are touched as a part of the overall nursing procedure. You touch a patient when you take his temperature, blood pressure, give an injection or bed-bath. In fact, there is no way to practice nursing without touching. And how you handle—touch—your patient says a great deal about the way you feel toward him and his illness. The nurse who is reluctant to squeeze the hand of an aphasic patient may have no aversion to that patient, but merely an upbringing that makes touching situations difficult. Unfortunately, the patient has no way of knowing, and is only aware of her aversion.

Tactile communication is transitory, it lasts only while it is being done. It is also reciprocal; nurse and patient touch each other. Touch is the most personal of our senses because it brings two human beings into a close relationship. It is the most basic and primitive of the senses; the infant uses touch to explore its world, and while still a fetus, responds to the vibrations of the mother's heartbeat. Our first contact with life is through touch. The newborn feels the obstetrician's hands, reacts to the feel of touch during rocking, soothing, bathing, and feeding. The baby's first cry is usually silenced when he is placed on his mother's belly and experiences her warm comfort. Our first comfort in life comes from touch—and usually our last, since touch may communicate with the comatose, dying patient when words have no way of breaking through.

Through touch, the whiskers of a cat give information necessary for its life. In man, the receptors for touch are in the skin. Some see the skin as having a mind; others, as a cloak that covers us all over. It is the oldest and the most sensitive of our organs, the first medium of communication and our most efficient protector. Next to the brain, the skin is perhaps the most important of all organ systems, and the sense most closely associated with the skin is the sense of touch.

When a child touches a hot, cold, or rough object, he will withdraw because of pain. He learns to associate these objects as signs of pain, and he avoids them and later responds symbolically to the words: hot, cold, rough. If a pediatric patient perceives roughness in a nurse, he may refuse to talk to the next nurse because she symbolizes pain.

Touch contacts are so vital to human development that children will fail to grow and to mature without them. A total deprivation of touching leads to cachexia in some children, which can cause death or retardation, while other children given a scant ration of physical affection grow into destructive, violent adults. The importance of touch to human beings cannot be stressed too much, and caring touch contacts are necessary to the therapeutic environment. It is vital that student nurses recognize the dynamic force of touch within the interpersonal relationship and develop sensitivity to it.

Sharon L. Roberts writes about the importance of touch to the hospitalized adult in her text *Behavioral Concepts and the Critically Ill Patient:*

> In today's highly technical hospital environment, dominated by machines, the patient loses precedence to the machines. The patient then experiences technological deprivation. With technological deprivation comes emotional deprivation. For example, a patient in ICU may be surrounded by various pieces of equipment: a cardioscope, a chest tube and gomco station, IVs and a respirator. (As the nurse comes to the patient's bed, she approaches his equipment first; when the equipment is checked, she then looks at the patient.) This is a correct nursing response: she must run rhythm strips, check dial settings, rate of IV solution, and carry out other procedures. After gathering her data, the nurse will move toward her patient and, possibly, touch him, but she has given more nursing care time to the various machines than to her patient. The nurse cannot be faulted for this because she must fill the squares on her patient's chart with numbers and words at the designated time. She has patient responsibilities, her time is limited, she must gather her data and move on to the next patient. Day nurses must put all their data in order before the parade of doctors and technicians begins.
>
> Sometimes machines make the data collection too easy. The nurse may begin to rely on the machines for data instead of her own eyes and judgment. Reliance on machines diminishes the amount of sensory input from touch. When the nurse limits her touching to the patient's equipment, the patient experiences emotional deprivation.[4]

Tactile communication belongs to man's inner world, even as it belongs to his outer world. Patients who have no apparent verbal capacity can usually feel a gentle touch and understand its message of caring interest.

Unfortunately, many adults have mixed feelings about touch. Some carry childhood taboos into adulthood, whereas others see tactile contact as an invasion of their privacy or are bothered by feelings of embarrassment and inferiority. Understanding our own feelings will help us empathize with our patients' responses to touch.

Students often find that role playing can be a helpful means of insight. In a classroom setting, this role playing can be between students. Each may take a turn at acting out the symptoms. One student may pace the floor, another weep, and a third retreat into silent staring as they act out the patient's response to a scheduled amputation. The audience will look for cues to which the patient-role player is receptive and gauge the nurse-role player's reaction. What cues did she respond to? Would her response ease your own anxiety?

Although touch may be accompanied by words, it is frequently more meaningful when performed without words. There are times when the best expression of empathy is in nonverbal touch. For instance, a young primipara who had given birth to a dead baby was severely traumatized. The nurse caring for her had a problem in dealing with her own sorrow for what this mother had to endure. Realizing that the mother had to grieve, the nurse listened as the patient poured out her feelings. It was by touching— by holding her hand, laying a cold cloth on her forehead, and rubbing her sore back —that the nurse communicated that she cared. All that she did with touch said how much she wanted to help. This nurse subordinated her own feelings of sorrow. She was free to devote her energy to the best interests of her patient.

Some physical symptoms can best be evaluated by touch, such as determining the rate, rhythm, and strength of the pulse. Circulatory disturbances in the extremities may be checked by touching both feet or both hands. Information about the dampness of a patient's clothing from perspiration, drainage, or elimination can sometimes come only through the fingertips. Palpation may disclose fluid in the tissues or locate an enlargement of an organ, such as the liver, or a tumor.

The nurse's sensitive touch will find snarls in the patient's hair and avoid unnecessary pulling during combing. The same hands will find and smooth away wrinkles underneath the patient and fluff up the pillow to a desired softness. Even the temperature of the bath is most frequently determined by putting one's hands in the water.

Touch tells us a great deal about the patient's physical state, and it also can convey information about his emotional well-being, since he transmits the realities of his own world more accurately nonverbally than verbally.

A patient may reach out to grasp the nurse's hand, seeking comfort and reassurance through the sense of touch. The positive feelings of sympathy, reassurance, understanding, and compassion are transmitted through touch—just as are the negative feelings of anger, hostility, and fear. To be truly therapeutic, tactile communication must be used at the appropriate time and place. Each person considers a certain amount of space around him as private, and touch can be seen as an invasion of that privacy unless it is desired by each person. Touch must be used at the right time and in the right way; otherwise misinterpretation of the message will occur.

The use of touch by people is not limited to communication. It is also used as a means of becoming familiar with the environment. Children fondle a new toy, examine every inch of it with their fingers, and clutch it tightly until it has become familiar. Adult patients exhibit the same kind of touch exploration when they pat the hospital bed or run their fingers up and down its raised safety bars. The patient's need to keep in touch with his environment is real, and the observant nurse will be aware that the patient's touch behavior has significance. A patient who is constantly touching a certain area of his body might be experiencing pain, unusual sensations, or fear that this part of his body is in danger.

It is through touch that we become oriented to the spatial dimensions of our world. It is through touch that we really feel the emotions of others. Touch was considered so powerful in the past that it was used as a therapeutic tool, and cures were attempted by the "laying on-of-hands." This act consisted simply of placing the hands on or near the body of an ill person in an attempt to heal that person.

Modern nurses still have much to learn about the significance of touch as an essential component of nursing care. There is a special need to recognize the therapeutic properties of touch, and a further need for nursing research and implementation in this area.

Facial Expressions

Facial expressions can reinforce our words or wipe them out completely. A smile, a frown, a raised eyebrow, compressed lips, lowered eyelids, eyes that will not meet ours —all these convey emotional states. The face is a strong communicator; it provides us with nonverbal feedback from others as we speak to them. The eyebrow raised in disbelief, the frown, the nervous chewing of the lip—these signs tell us how the other person is reacting to what we are saying. We pay a great deal of attention, usually on the subconcious level, to these facial cues and are apt to pick up quickly any discrepancy between facial cue and verbal symbol.

Although we are able to pick up facial cues and sense their meaning on an undefined level of consciousness, this general awareness may not be sufficient in the nursing-care situation. Delivery of quality nursing care depends on understanding and meeting the patients' needs. When some of those needs are expressed nonverbally through facial expression, nurses are justified in asking for more concrete guidelines in interpreting facial cues.

Over one hundred years ago, Charles Darwin[5] wrote that facial expressions of emotion are universal, not learned differently in each culture. Darwin's theory was not universally accepted, and many writers since his time have disagreed with it. Paul Ekman and Wallace Friesen in *Unmasking the Face*[6] agree with Darwin's theory. In their own research, they discovered what they believe to be "consistent and conclusive evidence that accurate judgments of facial expression can be made." Their experiments dealt basically with the six emotions of happiness, sadness, surprise, fear, anger, and disgust. Ekman and Friesen described the facial cues of each of the six emotions as follows:

1. Surprise is the briefest emotion . . . it doesn't linger. . . . In surprise, the eyebrows appear curved and high, the skin below the brow is lifted. The surprise brow is usually joined by wide open eyes and dropped jaw.

2. People fear harm. The fear may be physical or psychological or both. . . . There is a distinctive appearance in each of the three main facial areas during fear. The eyebrows are raised and drawn together; the eyes are open, the lower lid is tensed, and the lips are stretched back.

3. Disgust is a feeling of aversion . . . The most important clues to disgust are manifested in the mouth and nose and to a lesser extent in the lower eyelids and eyebrow. The upper lip is raised, while the lower lip may be raised or lowered, the nose is wrinkled, the lower eyelids are pushed up, and the eyebrow is lowered.

4. Anger is probably the most dangerous emotion. . . . Although there are distinctive changes in each of the three facial areas during anger, unless changes occur in all three areas, it is not clear whether or not a person is actually angry. The eyebrows are lowered and drawn together, the eyelids are tensed, and the eye appears to stare in a hard fashion. The lips are either tightly pressed together or parted in a square shape.

5. Happiness is the emotion most people want to experience. . . . Happiness is shown in the lower face and lower eyelids. Corners of the mouth are drawn back and up. The mouth may or may not be parted, with teeth exposed or not. A wrinkle (the nasolabial fold) runs down from the nose to the outer edge beyond the lip corners. The cheeks are raised. The lower eyelid shows wrinkles below it, and may be raised but not tense. Crows'-feet wrinkles go outward from the outer corners of the eyes.

6. In sadness your suffering is muted . . . In its most extreme form, there may be no facial clue to sadness other than the loss of muscle tone in the face. There is a distinctive appearance in each of the three facial areas during sadness. The inner corner of the upper eyelid is drawn up, and the lower eyelid may appear raised. The corners of the lips are drawn down, or the lips appear to tremble.

Many researchers disagree with Ekman and Friesen. They believe that it is difficult to evaluate facial cues accurately without contextual input. Until more concrete evidence is agreed upon, the Ekman and Friesen category of facial expression should be used only as a guide in relationship to other known aspects of the patient's condition.

Gestures

We often hide our real feelings when we write or talk, revealing them in subtle behaviors as gestures. Gestures frequently accompany speech, and we are seldom aware of just how much gesturing we do. A patient moving restlessly in bed, a child squirming, someone tapping his fingers—all of these behaviors tell the patient's story, and as nurses we must become skilled in interpreting these gestures if we are to learn how the patient really experiences his world. Emotions do manifest themselves physically. The tension created by anxiety, for example, can cause tachycardia, elevated blood pressure, excessive perspiration, and, in some cases, diarrhea—all of which are potentially dangerous to the recuperating patient. Yet, the early signs of anxiety are there for us to see. They can be most clearly observed in the patient's gestures: restlessness, pacing, increased movement of the extremities, disorientation, and other nonverbal clues.

Empathy and Mutual Trust

We speak of empathy and relating one-to-one as vital humanistic goals. Actually, we have to mean relating on a one-to-one basis effectively, since the relationship is already one-to-one. There is no other way to perform many nursing tasks. No system has been devised for giving a remote control enema. You deal with your patients in a very personal way. When you approach them with empathy, you create an environment that will enable them to respond best to the actual nursing procedure. Frightening, angering, bullying, or traumatizing your patients does little to enhance their recuperation.

Empathy is the ability of one person to penetrate the covert thoughts and feelings of another and to interpret them as if they were his own without losing his identity. In nursing, this definition can be carried to the point of saying that empathetic communication is associated with the nurse's sincerity, genuine liking of her patient, her sensitive understanding of that patient's private world, and her ability to communicate these feelings to the patient.

Communication barriers, on the other hand, are obstructions that hamper and impede interaction between patient and nurse. They result because of misunderstanding, fear, anxiety, fatigue, and psychological blindness. In his study, *Some Barriers to Communications,* James K. Skipper, Jr., points out that "patients were in a sense fearful of the power and the authority of the nurse, and intimidated in the presence of the doctor."[7] Therefore, the communication process was at least partially blocked. Is it any wonder that messages are often not received as sent, or are misinterpreted. Meaning is the heart of any communication, and the nurse must be aware of what she reflects in her nonverbal levels in order for the correct meaning to be transmitted to the patient.

Mutual trust follows empathy. The patient should trust the nurse, and the nurse must risk disclosure of her own individuality if that trust is going to occur. This disclosure does not mean telling the patient about your own personal problems, but rather revealing the humane and human aspects of your personality.

Silence

"Speech is of time, silence is of eternity." But how easy speech is to handle in comparison to silence. Yet just as there is positive and negative verbal communication, there is positive and negative silence. In silence, people may express feelings ranging from empathy and love to resentment and hostility. Silence can be punishing and can infer rejection, such as silence accompanied by the direct gaze that one person gives to another, which seems to say: "You disappoint me," or "Did you do it wrong again?" There is another kind of silence that communicates affection, and we see this with young lovers who frequently sit silently gazing at one another. Silence does have range, and when this is understood it becomes less threatening.

It is necessary to be silent if we wish to listen to another person. Many people are not good listeners for this reason. They are uncomfortable when they are not speaking and cannot wait for the other person to finish so they can talk again. Dominick Barbara describes the effective listener as one who uses silence with as much eagerness as he uses talk.[8]

A chattering nurse can be very unnerving to the patient. Physiologically, there are times when the patient needs silence. This is one of the reasons "quiet zones" exist in our hospitals.

When silence is used constructively, nurses can weave stronger ties with patients. Recently, a nurse being interviewed described the following scene:

> My patient had expired, and the family came to view their loved one for the last time in the hospital. I greeted them without words and stood silently with them at the bedside. The silence seemed comforting. It allowed us all time to adapt and to cope with our feelings. By means of silent contemplation, I was able to view the deceased as he actually was, and the family was able to accept their loss gradually in the privacy of their own thoughts.

Active Listening

Active listening is almost, but not quite, part of silence. It is an active process, while silence is passive. Active listening requires understanding, skill, patience, and perseverance. Encouraging the patient to express himself will not be helpful if he senses that you are not listening. Attentive listening is another way of saying active listening. It refers to the attitude of the nurse; it means that she is ready to hear what the patient wants to say and will endeavor to understand his situation without argument, interruption, or judgment.

Active listening requires concentration, since you must listen for the meaning of the words. A voluntary effort is needed to understand what is being said. This is most. successfully achieved when there is a definite goal. Most of us have had the experience of being in a class and finding to our discomfort that we were not listening when a question was specifically directed toward us. If we have the purpose of listening in mind, what we hear will capture our attention—we begin to think, to listen actively and enthusiastically. When the nurse's manner reflects enthusiasm, she responds to the patient. The communication takes on meaning. The nurse can lean forward when the patient says something important, nod in agreement, and add a word here and there to enhance the conversation. People feel important and respected when they are listened to.

We acquire good listening habits by first learning to keep quiet. This means not interrupting the patient. Sometimes people pause to clarify their thinking or to search for a word. The nurse should refrain from rephrasing the patient's last sentence or supplying the word she thinks the patient is looking for. Instead, she should use the silent pause to think through what the patient has said. She should never correct, interrupt, or disagree because this would defeat her purpose, which is to understand her patient's need, and often his greatest need is for someone to listen to him.

Ordinarily, our hearing is only "half on," or passive, but when we make a conscious effort it becomes active. What we do with the listening time determines whether we are good or poor listeners. Good listening is an essential ingredient for providing nursing care of good quality. Although most nurses are aware of the need to listen, patients still sometimes report, "The nurse was too busy to listen." Some nurses only half listen or do not listen at all.

Territoriality

The term "territoriality" is frequently used in behavioral studies. It denotes the human tendency to stake out personal territory, just as animals do. The lion patrols his hunting area to keep others out; by extension, we see evidence of human territoriality all around us. At home, we speak of mother's kitchen, dad's garage, Uncle Joe's easy chair, and my TV. As a group, we cheer for our team, vote for our candidate, and worship in our church. The concept of territoriality includes space and things that we mark off as belonging primarily to us.

When a patient is checked into the hospital, territorial things and space are left behind. The day before he checks into the hospital, he has a clear identity, which is reinforced by all of his territorial surroundings. Suddenly, the night before surgery he finds himself in unfamiliar, often frightening surroundings, wearing an embarrassing hospital gown. He was probably cautioned to leave his wallet, jewelry, and credit cards at home. There is no territorial reinforcement. He has ceased to be John Jones, the most successful plumber in East Hamden, Ohio. He has become, instead, Dr. Smith's gallbladder case. It is all routine for us, but it is not for him. A little empathy for his nervousness might go a long way toward helping him through the next day's ordeal.

Long-term patients have special problems in relating to their hospital environment. For example, an elderly patient in a skilled nursing facility suddenly lost her husband. She mourned terribly and developed the habit of opening a small box of memorabilia kept in her bedside stand, strewing the contents all over her bed—pictures, bits of ribbon, old letters, and other souvenirs. One of the staff nurses would catch her, scold the patient for being so messy, carefully pack everything into the box and pop it back into the night stand. The elderly lady would cry and dig the box out again as soon as the nurse's back was turned. The nurse did not recognize that the box of memorabilia was the old woman's last tie with her territory—with all that was her life.

Flowers are allowed, even encouraged, because they brighten up the room and create a more alive and less sterile atmosphere. Some hospitals have cork boards in the room where get-well cards can be tacked up for the patient to see. A young nurse was upset over the depression of an elderly patient. In a conversation with his daughter, she learned that he was terribly fond of his grandchildren. She asked the daughter to bring pictures of the children, then tacked the pictures on the cork board. The patient was delighted, began eating better and, in general, exhibited a much improved state of mind.

While it is true that we cannot move Uncle Joe's easy chair into his hospital room, we can do small things that make the patient feel more at home. Such touches may be as important to his overall progress as the room's cleanliness and temperature control. The patient, in the course of his recovery, will probably be subject to many unpleasant, painful, and frightening procedures; let us not compound these with any unnecessary trauma.

Territories can be marked off and are visible to others. Another dimension of proxemics, however, is not as easy to identify. Personal space is invisible and mobile. It is the spatial area around our bodies that we consider personal. The distances of personal space will vary from individual to individual. Some people become uneasy at distances of several feet; others are comfortable at an intimate distance. Generally speaking, intimate distance is from zero to about twenty-four inches, a proximity which brings two people into close physical contact. Proximity influences communication; when two people are very close, they become aware of each other's physical presence. There is likely to be very little verbalization. Touch conveys many of the messages we normally verbalize in close body contact, and only by narrowing the distance are such touching behaviors as holding, hugging, grasping, and stroking possible.

Some people use their personal space as a protection and are threatened when it is invaded. We have all observed two-party conversations where one person moves in very close—almost nose-to-nose—to make his point. The other person often sees this as an invasion of his personal space and responds by pulling his head back. If this first nonverbal cue is not received, he may even step back and away.

Nurses, because of the procedures they perform, are involved with patients at intimate distances. Many patients will be uncomfortable with this necessary closeness; nurses can ease the patient's anxiety by paying special attention to their facial expressions and touching contacts, which should convey a sense of cheerful consideration and gentleness.

Time

Time is the vehicle for both verbal and nonverbal communication. Time is not traditionally included in nonverbal studies because time is neither spatial nor behavioral. But all behaviors do take place within the dimension of time. Time is involved when the nurse sits quietly by the bedside of a dying patient, or when she pauses to give a sick child extra attention. In the nursing environment, time becomes a component of communication. Time spent with a patient when no procedure is being performed communicates interest and caring to the patient. The commitment of time becomes, in itself, communication.

In busy hospitals where the patient census is high, time becomes critical, but the caring nurse will still attempt to utilize her time to meet the patient's needs. The reader will see later how a busy director of nurses in a skilled nursing facility always made the time to greet and chat with her patients.

Nurses who spend unsolicited time with patients demonstrate, nonverbally, their commitment to the patient. They also enhance their own efficiency and ability to manage time. A visit with the patient provides an excellent opportunity for observation; the patient's present needs can be assessed, his future needs discussed and anticipated. Frequently, an anticipated need can be met immediately, decreasing the possibility that it will become critical just when the day is the busiest and the entire callboard looks like the lights of Broadway on opening night.

Nonverbal Dynamics

Touch, facial expression, body movement, gestures, empathy, trust, and environment are all dimensions of nonverbal communication. They are phases of a subject that is of tremendous importance in the patient-centered approach to nursing. Nonverbal communication is a nursing skill, learnable and teachable, just as any of the other nursing skills are. Most of what we learn in nursing is concerned with the efficacy and the success of a procedure. Nonverbal communication can be used as a tool for creating the environment in which the well-learned and well-executed procedure will have the best therapeutic value.

So far, we have discussed, in general terms, what components are involved and how nonverbal communication can be of overall benefit to you and to your patient. The following material will be more specific and deal with definite areas and procedures for nonverbal communication in nursing.

2

Confused Communication
Clarified

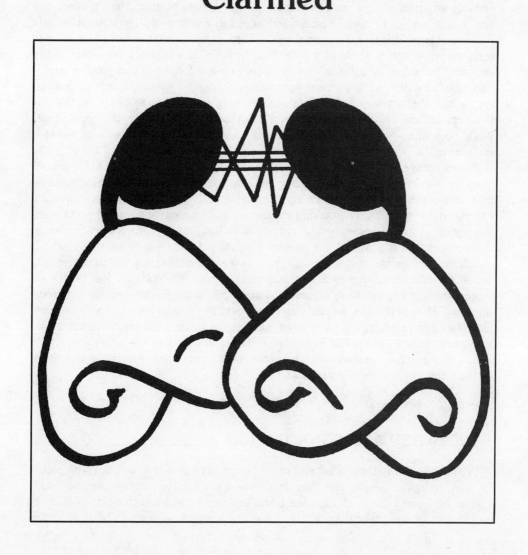

In view of the rapidly advancing technology in this century, it is quite possible that some day someone will invent a mechanical communication device, and instrument so sensitive it could receive and transmit, unerringly, the true spirit, intent, and context of each verbal and nonverbal message. But until this wonder materializes, we will have to be satisfied with our somewhat less than perfect human mechanisms. Unfortunately for the poor nursing student trying to learn therapeutic communication, there is no fail-proof method of relating to patient groups. We can label the groups A, B, C, and come up with some generalizations. We can categorize elderly patients in group C and note that they are all facing the last stage of life, with its concurrent deterioration of physical and mental capabilities. Patients in group C would exhibit some of the same behaviors, so it would be very easy to assume that we could use a behavioral set in relating to them. This would be an extremely shortsighted view. Patients are people first and patients second, and each brings his own uniqueness into the nursing care situation.

With group C again in mind, a second and equally erroneous assumption could be made. We could assume that a behavioral set would be viable if it were based on one or more group subcategories. The first subcategory could be ethnic background, and you would tune in to specific behavioral expectations from elderly Italians, elderly Chinese, elderly Chicanos, and so on, and, in turn, program your verbal and nonverbal behavior with them in terms of a prescribed formula. It would not work even if you continued to add subcategory after subcategory covering cultural background, education, marital status, socioeconomic environment, religion, politics, sports preference, etc. In fact, the only way such a system of grouping would work would be to continue to categorize and cross-reference three billion times, because that is the approximate world population—a group figure, but made up of all the individuals in the world—each seeing the world with his own vision.

Nurses are as equally unique and imperfectly human as their patients. That ingenious inventor who in an age yet to come may develop the perfect communication machine may also come up with a perfect nursing machine. It might look something like a computerized iron lung. The nursing machine would transmit and receive verbal messages with complete accuracy and carry out skilled nursing procedures flawlessly. When the patient is admitted, the physician would put him into the nursing machine, punch the appropriate computer mix, then return at the end of the prescribed hospitalization to either discharge or bury his patient. There would be no lost charts, no inaccurate observations, no misunderstood messages, no confusion. The nursing procedures would be perfection, but nursing care would be nil. Machines cannot care, only imperfect human beings can care, listen, provide the warmth of a gentle touch, empathize, and create a therapeutic environment. So let us hope that the future genius who would create such a machine is very far in the future, and return to the present problem of the imperfectable art of communication.

DENOTATION AND CONNOTATION

We have seen why there is not and never can be any one way to interact with people or with groups of people. But that does not mean that basic communication skills cannot be learned and with experience and practice be adapted to meet a variety of situations that will make the practice of nursing more effective. Our ability to understand verbal messages is influenced by other factors, and the most important of these is the concurrent nonverbal communication. The person who really understands this will use nonverbal cues to reinforce the spoken word, to clarify the confusion that always results, to a large or to a small degree, when two people try to talk to each other. We do confuse each other with our words because a word may have several denotations and a wide variety of individual connotations. A young French student who was studying English went to his instructor for clarification of the word "fast," which he found very confusing.

"I cannot understand this word," he began. "You say: I ran fast and you say: a young lady with loose morals is fast. Also, colors that do not fade are fast. I just read in my book about an old man who was fast asleep and, then, to my horror, when one doesn't eat all day, you say it is because of his fast. So, please tell me what fast means."

The student was confused over the denotation of fast. In each example that he presented, fast was used correctly in accordance with its definition, but it was difficult for the student to accept so many meanings for one word. The confusion multiplies rapidly when we add connotation, which is the associative implication of a word. Words simply defined are messages. If a word has one connotation to the sender and another to the receiver, the message is lost.

A nursing colleague told us an experience she had while vacationing in Ireland:

... It was raining quite heavily, so I decided to give a lift to a young girl who was hitchhiking on the road. She was pleasant enough, and we chatted for ten minutes or so about this and that. I was enjoying the lovely lilt of her brogue, and she didn't seem to be having too much trouble understanding my midwestern twang. Suddenly, she turned to me and said, "You're very plain."

Well, my first instinct was to stop the car and put her out, rain or no rain. Here I was nice enough to give her a lift and she insults me. Talk about nonverbal behavior, I didn't say anything but I gripped the steering wheel tightly and stared into the rain.

After I cooled down, we talked again and I soon learned that she meant I spoke clearly and she had no trouble understanding me, and we had a good laugh when I explained that back home plain meant downright homely.

The connotation of plain to the young Irish girl was clear; it meant easy to understand. She had never heard it used to describe an unattractive person. The nurse was used to hearing the word plain in terms of homeliness, so the message that was sent as a compliment was received as an insult.

Our ability to understand verbal messages is not based solely on denotation and connotation. It is influenced by additional factors; nonverbal communication is one of the more important of these, but attitude, knowledge, social background, culture, and physical and mental state are additional considerations. In communicating, we attempt to send a message to another person. Generally we know whether or not the message has been received correctly because of the feedback from that other person. Feedback usually tells us that the message has been understood or misunderstood. If it has not been received as sent, we try again and modify, rephrase, or use some other means of getting through. The heart of the communication, the message, must pass from one person to another through uncharted, nonformulated, undefined psychic space. This journey begins in the private world of one human being and ends in the private world of another.

Communication problems are not limited to the medical field. A rather common sight in business offices is a plaque stating, "I know you think you understand what you thought I said . . ." An in-office communication breakdown does present a serious business problem, but this problem really cannot be viewed in the same context as communication in the nursing situation. Communication is a nursing responsibility, since it is a means of filling the patient's needs. There is no nursing procedure that is not accompanied by some form of communication—verbal or nonverbal—and each message does have an impact on the patient. Through good communicative skills, we demonstrate to the patient that we are concerned with his welfare; therefore, nursing communications become therapeutic in nature.

THERAPEUTIC NONVERBAL COMMUNICATION _____

The word "therapeutic" means to heal or to cure, and therapeutic communication is directed toward easing the patient's condition and environment. Therapeutic communication takes planning, but planning should not be confused with artificiality or contrivance. Any action that is insincere will be spotted by the patient and come across as phony. The first rule of therapeutic communication is to be genuine, to be yourself. Nonverbal communication, especially, will not be effective unless it is real and expresses your true feelings. By planned communication, we mean communication that is goal directed and aimed toward specifics in the patient-care plan. Patient-care goals can vary from one nursing situation to another. In a skilled nursing facility, an illustrative goal might be the rehabilitation of a CVA (cerebral vascular accident) patient. In this situation, the primary aim is for the patient to feed himself. Therapeutic communication would be planned around this goal. Verbally, the nurse would encourage the patient to feed himself, reinforce his progress, and offer support when things were not going well, saying such things as: "You're doing just fine . . . You've improved so much just this last week . . . Don't be upset, we all have days when it seems that we are not making much progress . . ." So far, so good! However, without the strong support of nonverbal interactions, the rehabilitative goal will not be met. If the nurse appears disgusted as she cleans the patient up after an unsuccessful feeding attempt or handles his soiled linens gingerly, her behavior is not reinforcing. It is saying: "You're not doing fine . . . I see no progress . . . You can't even perform a simple task that any bright two-year old is capable of doing . . ."

The patient will become confused. The nurse is saying one thing, but her behavior is not expressing the feeling and intent of her words. In fact, her behavior is expressing the exact opposite. The patient will accept her behavior as the real truth and may even begin to view himself as a hopeless case. Words alone do not constitute therapeutic communication. The patient may think that the words are rote learned by all nurses and delivered to all patients as perfunctorily as the evening medications.

When the patient gives up and refuses to try to feed himself, the nurse will become confused. She will probably report, at the next staffing, that she has consistently used verbal reinforcement with the patient, is unable to understand his refusal to feed himself, and can only assume that he is more severely brain damaged than originally diagnosed. This misinterpretation of the facts could lead to misdirected therapy.

Therapeutic communication consists of effective messages that are understood. The message contains both verbal and nonverbal components. The verbal component should be stated simply and clearly. The nonverbal component should express the intent and the feeling of the message. In the above illustration, the nurse's verbal component was lost because her behavior was incongruent.

NURSING DATA

Good nursing care is based on accurate data: (1) medical information, which has been established through physical examinations, laboratory work, X-rays, and so on; (2) nursing observations—perception of the patient's nonverbal behavior; (3) verbal exchanges that provide information on the patient's physical and emotional state.

Patients generally tell us about their true state by their behavior, even when their words express what they think they should say. A postsurgical patient refused a Demerol injection, saying: "It's not bad at all. I just don't give in to a little pain. I've never even taken an aspirin in my whole life." An aide who entered the patient's room unexpectedly with fresh water sometime later reported that the patient was moaning and restless. The behavior expressed the patient's real state. He did have pain. His words may have been influenced by a familial background in which "only cowards gave in to pain." Patients' immediate needs must be met, and these needs are usually expressed more clearly through nonverbal cues than they are through words. Patients tell us about their real world through their behaviors. We must use all of our senses to interpret the nonverbal cues and relate the behavior to the situation. We must look for harmony or disharmony of behaviors.

The information we receive from patients must be clear. Therapeutic communication depends on clarity. Well-planned nursing care also depends on clarity. Therefore, we must understand what our patients are saying, and this is not always easy. Some patients are intimidated, difficult to understand, hesitant, confused, and reluctant to express themselves. Sometimes, we must repeat a question several times, rephrase it, and paraphrase it until we do have all the necessary information and understand it clearly. Information gaps impede nursing care. For example, when questioned, the patient responds that he has a headache "all the time." Does he really mean that his head hurts all day and all night? Is the pain really constant? The information, as stated, is incomplete. The nurse might need to rephrase her question. "Are there times during the day," she asks, "when the headache is less severe . . . more severe?" With careful questioning, she can fill in the informational gaps as she learns and records that the patient has prolonged headaches—most severe in the morning and often accompanied by nausea . . . the pain abates mid-day leaving an aura of soreness, with intense pain experienced again in the evening.

Patients' interviews will be facilitated by nonverbal communication. Active listening helps clarify communication by focusing our attention on the patient. As we concentrate on what he has to say, we come to understand his realities. We are better able to put aside our own attitudes and assumptions and concentrate on his perception as he expresses it to us verbally and nonverbally. Attention is frequently a two-way street, and because we listen to what the patient is saying, he, in turn, will pay more attention when it is his turn to listen.

Silence invites response and gives the patient time to formulate an answer. During silence, the nurse will have time to evaluate the data and assess the patient's anxiety level. Anxiety is a form of stress. Stress blocks communication. Silent periods allow the nurse to identify anxiety and to intervene.

Facial expression, especially eye contact, and set of the mouth tell the patient that we are with him.

The nurse–patient relationship is made up of frequent interactions, both verbal and nonverbal. A skilled nurse will look for contradictions between the patient's verbal and nonverbal behavior and subtle behavioral changes. Words are often not what they seem and are sometimes used to camouflage what is actually felt.

Dean Barnlund describes nonverbal behavior as "an elaborate code that is written nowhere, known by none, and understood by all."[9] It conveys completely messages that are only partially transmitted verbally. Our nonverbal behaviors cannot be controlled with the accuracy that we can control our words; perhaps that is why they are more believable and more trusted.

MORE COMMUNICATION CONFUSERS

Generalization is another communication confuser. Sometimes, we form a generalization from a single nursing observation that may be untypical of the patient's usual behavior. We assume an attitude based on that faulty observation and then behave as if it were true. Subsequent interactions with the patient become invalid. The patient who refuses to feed himself is approached as "more brain damaged than originally diagnosed," when, in fact, he is merely confused by his nurse's mutually exclusive verbal and nonverbal cues. We choose not to answer a patient's light because he is always ringing the bell; another patient is given her medication last because she is a whiner and not in as much pain as she pretends to be. These could be erroneous assumptions based on faulty observations. They adversely affect communication and the quality of nursing care.

Attitudes influence our interactions with patients. Attitudes are not behaviors, they are perceptions which usually effect our behavior. Attitudes are often based on false assumptions. We stereotype an individual and approach him accordingly. This attitude may be the result of scanty or inaccurate information about him, or because of our experience with other people who seem similar to him. Mr. Jones is a lawyer from Tennessee. Last month, you cared for another lawyer from Tennessee who was a very difficult patient. Mr. Jones talks just like the previous patient, i.e., you approach Mr. Jones as if he were going to behave like the previous patient. You form a negative attitude toward Mr. Jones and that negative posture will influence all of your interactions with him.

Attitudes are communicated very quickly. The most effective attitude for a nurse is a positive one that does not stereotype patients because of inaccurate information or prior personal experiences. As nurses we can develop a positive attitude by being open, by accepting patients even when we do not totally understand or agree with their life styles. An open attitude can be related to the commitment we make in nursing, which calls for the care of all patients, not just the ones we can like and understand without effort.

Technical language causes additional confusion in nursing communications. The patient does not always understand what we are talking about. Even a phrase as simple as "vital sign" can cause confusion. A former patient confessed that she had been frightened when, immediately following surgery, the nurse came in every half-hour or so to take her vital signs. This patient was undergoing her first hospitalization, and although she had had blood pressure and pulse taken in her doctor's office, they had always been referred to as blood pressure and pulse. She recognized the procedure, but not the term vital sign. She knew vital meant life and assumed that the frequent checks were to see if she was still alive. Yet, "vital sign" is something we say as readily as "good morning," never thinking that a patient could be confused over what it means. The patient was awed by the nurse's authority and afraid to ask her about the procedure and its frequency. Communications in a medical setting are often blocked because the patient is intimidated by the power and authority of the nurse. Her professionalism blocks communication, the patient is afraid of angering her, or appearing silly and so does not ask: What does this procedure mean? Why is it being done? Is something wrong? Communication barriers, as we noted in Chapter 1, are obstructions that hamper communicative interaction on an interpersonal level, i.e., awe, fear, frustration, fatigue, environment, psychological blinders, and so forth.

FEEDBACK _____

The effectiveness of our communication is confirmed by feedback. Feedback regulates the back and forth transmission of messages. It helps us determine whether the message has been understood and, when it apparently has not, to try again. The reactions of the listener are the determining factors. Through feedback, we evaluate the interaction and make the appropriate correction. Feedback can be verbal: "I agree . . . I don't agree . . . Yes, I will . . . No, I won't." It can also be nonverbal: the raised eyebrow that may be saying, "I don't believe you"; the tightly pressed lips that are expressing anger; heads that bend toward you or away from you; twitching; turning away; and finger tapping are all forms of nonverbal feedback. It is difficult to explain the give and take of feedback. The process is very rapid. We transmit, receive, and modify almost instantaneously, frequently on a subconscious level, but always in response to the subtle behavioral cues of the other person.

Feedback can be positive or negative. We are not always willing to accept negative feedback. We block it, or recognize it, then discard it. We suspect the other person, and feel that he is out to get us. If the feedback is negative enough to be ego damaging, we may attack the other person verbally, or, in some cases, physically, and we may terminate the relationship, knowingly or unknowingly.

When giving feedback to a patient, we must be aware of his ego strengths, his emotional state. Appropriateness and timing are the prime considerations when giving patients negative feedback. Feedback is usually most effective when it is immediate, but sometimes it is more important to give the other person time to quiet his feelings. There is no sense overloading an already anxious, frightened, or suffering patient. Ideally, the negative message should be delivered at a time when it can be of value and when it can be understood. Any negative response should be descriptive rather than judgmental. Judgmental behavior almost always elicits defensive tactics that will furthur block and confuse communication. Other considerations for negative feedback are as follows:

1. Does the patient really want to hear it?
2. Does the patient trust you enough to believe you?
3. How comfortable is your relationship with the patient?
4. Will you have time to deal with the patient's response?

It is probably better to avoid negative feedback when you are unable to discern any beneficial outcome. Many patients are already overloaded with worries and problems and may not be able to cope successfully with any additional negativism. A comfortable nurse–patient relationship should exist, as well as a feeling of mutual trust, for without it the patient will block the feedback. Perhaps the most important point is that as a nurse you should never give a negative response when you do not have time to stay with the patient. If you "sock it to him" and leave, it will not have much therapeutic effect.

A thirty-two year old male patient with a newly diagnosed cardiac condition created havoc on his floor. He badgered and yelled at the young nurses, made disgusting sexual innuendos, and constantly ridiculed the hospital and its staff. The nurses dreaded going to his room and avoided it whenever possible, while the complaints piled up on the DN's desk. When she could take no more, the Director of Nurses confronted the patient with the accumulated negative feedback. She terminated the interview with the announcement: "Such behavior will no longer be tolerated," and left. The patient did not modify his behavior. He continued to be extremely difficult until the day of his discharge.

The DN's reaction was understandable, and perhaps justified, but the feedback did not result in a beneficial change. Perhaps if the Director of Nurses had approached the patient less judgmentally, established a comfortable relationship, and had remained with him, the feedback would have been more effective. The patient may have been reacting to the hospital staff out of anger caused by his physical condition rather than any real hostility toward the nurses. A more accepting attitude and a slightly greater investment of time may have enabled the patient to evaluate his behavior and find a less disrupting means of expressing his anger and frustration.

While negative feedback should be dispersed cautiously and sparingly, positive feedback should be spent lavishly. No opportunity should be missed to encourage the patient, to let him know that you like him, do not consider him or taking care of him a bother, that you are impressed by something he said or did, or that you agree with him. By and large, hospitals are not very reinforcing places for the patients. Your positive feedback and response encourage them and enable them to feel better about themselves and about you.

3

Talking to Your Patients without Words

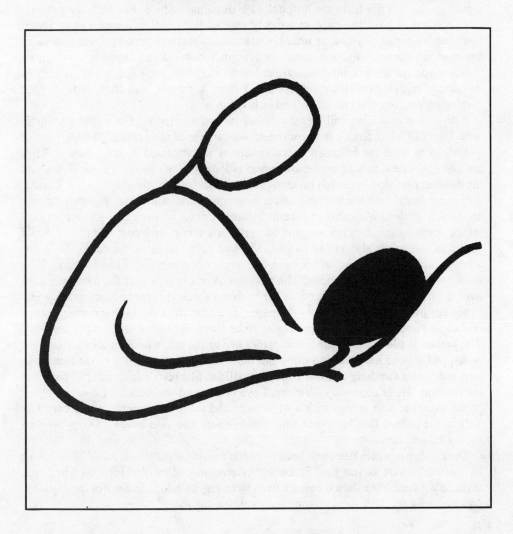

Anyone who has faced major surgery knows that it is not easy; even the most sophisticated among us has his moment of anxiety, apprehension, and just plain panic. Doctors and nurses are not immune and are often the worst patients, vocalizing their fears in criticism or complaints. It is understandable if medical personnel are difficult patients because they usually know the procedure and its prognosis equally as well as those who are caring for them do. However, there could be an additional explanation. Perhaps they are simply more familiar with the hospital environment, less intimidated, more apt to express verbally what other patients also feel but tell us only on a nonverbal level.

Some nurses are inclined to think that the patient is better off not knowing too much and ascribe to the old adage: "What you don't know can't hurt you." But it can. The patient does worry; anxiety is painful. He knows that the impending surgery is advisable or necessary. In most elective surgeries, his physician has assured him that it is a common procedure and that everything should go well. Common procedure? To whom? To the surgeon who has performed many similar operations, it is common. But, to the patient, it is a most uncommon procedure and, no matter how well everything should go, he will not leave the hospital with the same body he had when he entered. The patient will have to adjust to a newly scarred body that is minus a gallbladder, reproductive organ, thyroid, or breast. Occasionally there is the additional trauma of a permanent tracheotomy, or a surgically constructed stoma as a means of elimination.

When you nurse on a medical–surgical floor, surgeries soon become routine. You may care for five hysterectomies a week, twenty a month, and thousands in your nursing career, but the patient will have just the one.

With this in mind, we will create a rather typical admission. The patient, a thirty-seven year old white female with endometriosis, arrives at the hospital at 5:00 p.m. for surgery to be done the following morning. She is accompanied by her husband. They are told at the desk to wait until the business office calls their name; they sit down, and the minutes pass slowly as each pretends not to be nervous for the other's sake. Finally, they are ushered into the business office, where insurance and other financial matters are briskly settled. With that important business done, the patient is given a surgical release form authorizing her surgeon to perform a complete hysterectomy. The cold reality of the words shocks the patient. She had only talked to the doctor for a few minutes and had been upset at the time. She could not remember all he had said. Why hadn't she asked more questions? The business clerk explains that the form was standard, a formality. The patient notices her husband's worried face and not wanting him to see her own fear, quickly signs the paper. She tries to smile, saying nothing of her fear as he kisses her good-bye, promising to be there right after surgery the next day. The patient is silent as an aide accompanies her to the lab, where an identity bracelet is snapped around her wrist and urine and blood samples are taken. The lab technician does not notice anything unusual about the patient. She responds to his questions and instructions. He is unaware of her rapid eye blinks and the nervous fluttering of her hands. Another aide arrives with a wheelchair and takes the patient up to Room 520. Telling the patient that her nurse will soon be there, the aide leaves, closing the door tightly behind her.

Twenty-five minutes later, you head from the nursing station to Room 520, checking the patient's chart as you go: "Probable hysterectomy scheduled for 7:30 a.m.," you think to yourself. "She should be back from Recovery by noon, on her feet the day after, and home by the fifth day . . . routine." Routine to whom?

This will be your first and best opportunity to initiate a trusting, therapeutic relationship. This nervous patient is probably not going to verbalize her fears, but she will tell you something of her inner world by her unspoken behavior. Watch for the nervous laugh, forced cheerfulness, rapid eye blinks, lip biting, and the overflowing ashtray.

Once you realize that patients do have anxiety, you can help. A genuine smile, one that says I am prepared to like you and to care for you, is a good beginning. In a similar situation, the attending nurse could take a minute or two to explain the patient's new environment. She could show her how to work the call-button, the television, or tell her how to place outside calls, as the patient might be comforted by a call home sometime during her presurgery evening. These are small things done as you go about your routine. It takes no more time to say something to reinforce and to calm the patient, than it does to mention the warmth or coldness of the weather—which is not particularly important to her.

In interviewing a sampling of former surgical patients, we found that none had been asked the very good question: "Is this your first surgery?" It is surprising that this question is not asked more often, since it provides such an excellent opening for an explanation of preoperative procedures. When it is the patient's first surgery, you can say something like: "Maybe you'd like me to tell you about the schedule we'll be following with you tonight." If it is not the first surgery, you can still open your conversation along the same lines, saying: "You may remember that there were some special procedures that night before your last surgery, and we'll be doing some similar things tonight." Your discussion of the pre-op schedule will help the patient to cope with the evening's parade of enema bags, shaving kits, syringes, and so on.

Some hospitals have a policy of holding a "surgery class." A staff nurse meets with patients scheduled for surgery to discuss the hospital's program. The recovery area, postsurgical self-help, pain medication, and visiting schedules are outlined; then patients are encouraged to ask questions. This is basically a sound idea, since understanding should alleviate anxiety. However, patients who were recently interviewed have mixed feelings about the surgery class. The nurse who conducts the meeting is not seen again by many of the patients, so unless the entire nursing staff is aware of the orientation and willing to follow through, the purpose is lost. One patient spoke on the lack of follow-through.

> I was to have a thyroidectomy, and my doctor told me I would not be able to speak audibly for a day or two. I had been in that hospital before and knew that they had an intercom call system. When you rang, they asked you what you needed rather than just coming to the room. I mentioned this to the nurse who was conducting the class, saying that I was very much afraid that I would not be heard or understood. She assured me that my light was tagged, the nurses would know I couldn't speak, and would come directly to my room when the bell rang. But it sure didn't happen that way.

> The afternoon of my surgery, while I was alone in my room still hooked up to the intravenous bottle, I noticed fresh blood all over my bandages. I rang, but whoever answered just kept asking me to speak up and finally disconnected me. Nobody came to my room. I really thought that I was just going to lie there helplessly and bleed to death.

> After a while a nurse came to take my temperature, saw what was happening, and called my doctor. Things sure didn't go the way I was told they would in surgery class.

This patient exhibited a great deal of resentment in relating her story. For her, surgery class had been a farce because there was no staff follow-through. Someone obviously forgot to tag her light; the aide or ward clerk who answered her was poorly trained, resulting in the patient's loss of confidence in the nursing staff's ability or willingness to help.

If you will not be on duty when your patient returns from surgery, mention this, adding that you will look in on her as soon as your shift begins. You might even tell her the name of the assigned nurse, or charge nurse, who will be on duty when she comes back from surgery.

Your verbal and nonverbal communication, done well, should leave the patient comfortable in her environment, confident of your skills and sincere interest. Anxiety and apprehension will not disappear completely, but will be lessened by the time she is ready for sleep.

Preoperative nonverbal communication is on a broad level. It is used to create trust, confidence, and a therapeutic environment. It is directed toward alleviating fear, rather than to specific communication problems that have resulted from the surgical procedure. Postsurgically, you may be relating nonverbally to the patient in a different manner. You will not be looking for the same cues in a tracheotomy patient as you will in a colostomy patient. While it is not possible, within the confines of this text, to list a nonverbal repetoire for all surgeries, it might be helpful to look at some of the problems faced by patients undergoing specific surgeries.

TRACHEOTOMY PATIENTS

A patient who has undergone a tracheotomy is a classic example of dynamic nonverbal interaction. After this surgery has been performed the patient cannot speak and must communicate solely on a nonverbal level. The first twenty-four hours after the operation, in which a surgical opening through the neck has been made, are vital. The insertion of the cannula (an indwelling tube) facilitates the evacuation of secretions to permit breathing, but it prevents the patient from speaking. Therefore, tracheotomy patients must respond nonverbally.

The skilled nurse who has a good understanding of nonverbal behavior is able to plan her communications to relieve the patient's anxiety and to create an atmosphere of confidence. Careful observation for complications is important. The tracheotomy patient is afraid of choking, of being unable to breathe. This fear is generally manifested in such nonverbal actions as pleading eyes, fidgeting hands, tremors, and facial grimaces. Other symptoms that the patient exhibits nonverbally following a tracheotomy are restlessness and excitement, increase in respiratory and pulse rates, headache, nausea and vomiting, and anorexia. Blood pressure may be normal, but, as air hunger increases, the blood pressure will fall, cyanosis will appear, and twitching of the muscles may occur. It is important that the "trach" nurse understand these nonverbal signs, for the life of the patient depends upon a proper interpretation of his actions.

The nurse, in addition to interpreting the patient's nonverbal actions, must be able to ease his fears. Each nursing procedure performed should be explained in the simplest terms, slowly. Understanding will tend to lessen the patient's anxiety. Anxiety is also reduced by touching the patient, by facial expressions that show confidence, by carrying out procedures skillfully and gently, never giving the impression of being rushed or apprehensive, and by allowing the patient time to grasp what is going to happen.

Most patients who have had a tracheotomy are fearful that the signal light will not work, that hospital personnel will not come quickly, that the nurse may not fully understand the procedure and the dangers involved with breathing or fearful that they will never be able to speak again. The patient has many fears, and all of them are transmitted on a nonverbal level.

The understanding nurse will explain the use of pencil and pad as a temporary means of communication and will reassure the patient that he will be able to speak and breathe after the tube is removed. He should be assisted to cough in order to clear secretions, and he should be assured of close supervision, which will minimize his distress.

Some patients fear sudden death as a result of asphyxiation, so the nurse must appear to be sure of what she is doing. One of the most important times for the patient to get confirmation on how well things are going is when the nurse is suctioning the trachea. At this time, the patient may look at the nurse's face to see what her eyes are saying and to feel from her touch what her fingertips are saying. How gentle is she? How hurried is she? The patient may be asking, nonverbally, with his eyes, "How am I doing, nurse? How am I really doing?"

The tracheotomy patient breathes through the trach, rather than through his nose. The nurse should not assume that he understands this. She should explain how the trach works and that the patient will be kept breathing without interruptions.

Fear is conveyed, nonverbally, in the messages that are sent by tracheotomy patients. It is to be hoped that these cues will be received by the nurse in time for her to offer reassurance. She should watch for telltale signs of distress, which are often pain, sadness, anger, or anxiety. The patient's eyes window the feelings that are underneath and will tell you what he is experiencing.

Silence can serve as a listening time, a time to hear fear, to hear trach sounds that tell you it is time to suction again. Silent communication on the part of the nurse will ease the distress of the troubled patient, and patients with tracheotomies may be the most troubled of all patients.

COLOSTOMIES AND ILEOSTOMIES

Colostomies and ileostomies are relatively common operations. An artificial opening (stoma) is brought through the abdominal wall to create a temporary or permanent opening for drainage. Ileostomies (surgical removal of all or part of the small intestine) are permanent. Colostomies (surgical removal of all or part of the large intestine) can be either permanent or temporary. Postoperatively, ileostomy and colostomy patients can resume their former life style. They do not face the same adjustments that an amputee, cancer, or cardiac patient faces. But the surgery does alter the means of bowel evacuation and, for many patients, this results in feelings of revulsion and extreme embarrassment. These feelings can be most acute in the hospital when the patient is confronted with a dressing change or with an irrigation. Most people are conditioned to think of fecal matter as dirty and disgusting. The patient has to cope with the surgery and with his new means of evacuation. Temporarily, he will need help in performing a very personal and private bodily function that he has been doing independently since the age of two or three. He is faced with fears and with questions that cannot always be asked verbally because of his embarrassment. Therefore, we must look for nonverbal cues that indicate the patient's thoughts. The nurse can, by her own nonverbal actions, help overcome the shame, doubt, and unanswered questions that tend to make adjustment so difficult for colostomy and ileostomy patients.

Your verbal assurance to the patient that he can lead a busy and a successful life just as he did before surgery is not enough. It is through your nonverbal actions during the patient's hospitalization that he will develop the confidence and the ultimate acceptance that will enable him to resume the fullest measure of his former life.

An empathetic attitude is vital, as it helps to relieve the patient's distress. A major psychological hurdle for the patient is seeing the stoma for the first time and observing while the nurse cares for it. There should be some explanation, at this point, of the operation and its function. You should approach the patient in a confident manner and proceed to carry out the procedure as simply as possible. It is a nursing responsibility to teach the patient how to care for himself. Progressively explain each procedure by verbal instruction and with nonverbal actions. The patient, as he recovers, should be encouraged to participate in these procedures until he can perform them independently.

The patient's embarrassment is very real, and he is usually unaware that there are no obvious signs that he has had a colostomy/ileostomy and that no one need know unless he tells them. The patient can be made to realize this and to understand that his surgery does not have to be a handicap. Your counseling can free the patient from needless doubts, fears, shame, and unanswered questions which, if ignored, will impede his recovery and psychological adjustment.

The psychological care of the enterostomaic patient may be more demanding than the physical care. This surgery produces tremendous emotional trauma and requires understanding by all who care for the patient. When empathetic nursing care is provided, the patient takes the first step toward developing social confidence. The second step is accomplished by carefully teaching the patient to care for and to control his colostomy or ileostomy. The nonverbal use of models and of diagrams can be most useful during this second phase.

The patient may have difficulty seeing the dressing changed and smelling the disagreeable odor, so it is essential that the nurse indicate her calm acceptance of this procedure. The patient will look at her face to see if she is concerned or revolted. The best way for the nurse to relate nonverbally to the patient is to be considerate about the way she does the irrigation, the way she controls odor and splashing, and the way she slowly and gently cleanses away any drainage.

Frequently, colostomy/ileostomy patients are middle-aged or older; many are frail, undernourished, and debilitated. Their response to the shock of the surgery and its aftereffects may be so severe that they hope to die.

A young nurse, in dealing with a colostomy patient, was disturbed by the patient's refusal to eat. She had recognized his sensitivity and had been extremely careful of her own facial expressions, conversation, and touch contacts when she cared for his colostomy. But on the fifth day after surgery, the patient suddenly refused dinner and continued to refuse food for three days. The entire staff was puzzled, since his appetite had been quite normal until that time.

The nurse suddenly remembered an incident that had occurred on the same day the patient had first refused food. An aide had answered his call-button to find that the colostomy bag had burst, spilling fecal matter all over the patient's fresh incision. The aide called for help, and the nurse recalled hurrying to the room, experiencing the overpowering odor as she entered. With the aide's help, the patient was gently cleaned and changed. The nurse put the incident out of her mind. Now, she began to think about that burst bag, the patient's reaction, his terrible embarrassment and the way he had apologized over and over. Could it be that the patient was so embarrassed he would rather starve than to risk a repeat performance?

Her first impulse was to rush to the patient's room and to tell him that he mustn't feel that way, but she hesitated. This was her first colostomy patient, and she realized there was a great deal she did not know and that her actions might influence the patient's self-image for a long time to come. She went to a telephone book, looked up the local colostomy association. Ten minutes later, armed with a handful of notes and some valuable insight into the patient's problem, she started her rounds. She went, first to the hospital pharmacy to pick up some guard pills for the patient's colostomy bag. Then she visited the dietician to discuss menus that would help to control the odor problem. Finally, she went to see her patient. He ate dinner that night and did not miss another meal throughout his hospitalization.

It is exceedingly important that a nurse be competent in her procedures and skills, as this nurse was, but it is equally important that she be aware of how the patient is affected by what has happened to him. Understanding is the key. In this illustration, the nurse was prepared to understand. She was able to empathize with her patient and to see how an incident not uncommon in nursing could be devastating to him. She also drew on outside sources for additional knowledge and sensitivity because she recognized that her personal experience with colostomy patients was limited. She did not go on an ego trip, assuming that because she was the nurse she knew everthing about the patient's physical and mental state. Two to five years of schooling cannot provide all the answers; an effective nurse continues to learn and to grow every day of her professional life and, as her own knowledge expands, she has more resources for helping others.

Colostomy patients look right at you, watching for your expressions. If they see the nurse's look of disgust, the nurse–patient relationship is ruined. It is a good idea to use a room deodorizer to control unpleasant odors, and the patient's room should be aired daily. If the patient is sensitive, try to deodorize when he is not in the room.

A student nurse who cared for a colostomy patient said, "The patient watches to see how you care for the stoma. If the nurse accepts it, then the patient will learn to accept it." Another student said, "I could always tell how the patient felt by noticing several things—whether his nose was dilated or constricted; if he cleared his throat often, he was nervous; sometimes, the patients gag but I know nurses never should, not even student nurses."

A particularly sensitive student recalled two cases by saying, "One patient refused care, saying, 'I don't want you to do it. I can learn how to do it myself; besides, it doesn't have to be done right now.' He was too embarrassed to let me do it and I think he was using denial because he couldn't accept having a colostomy."

The other patient's wife remained in the room, apparently wanting her husband to be completely dependent on her. She would not let anyone else near her husband's colostomy. She said it was her duty to care for him because she was his wife.

Some patients are embarrassed by the appearance of the stoma; others by the odor. Many find it distasteful when the stoma bubbles and gurgles. They may keep these feelings locked in in stony silence and express them only by swallowing hard, tensing their muscles, and staring hard at the ceiling, as if to block out the scene.

In an interview with a recent graduate nurse who is also an ileostomy patient, we asked if her decision to become a nurse was influenced by her own treatment. She replied that it definitely was: "It's not that I am going to do so much in the nursing profession, but I do think I can do a lot for patients who are going through the same thing I did. It's for that reason that I intend to take special training in enterostomy care." She went on to explain that she felt that the psychological recovery of the ileostomy patient was as important as the physical recovery. The physical recovery may even depend on the psychological adjustment.

> Body image is terribly important to us all, and people who have had their normal means of evacuation altered do have a difficult time adjusting. The road to both physical and psychological recovery begins in the hospital. We nurses must be concerned with the quality of the patient's continued life, just as we are concerned with saving his life.

She went on to say personally that, even with the best care, it had been difficult for her to adjust. She still hates the changes in her body caused by the surgery. But then she reminds herself that it was a life-saving procedure, gives herself a swift kick mentally and gets on with living. Her husband has been wonderful, just as warm and loving as before the surgery. Everyone is not so lucky, and she tells us of a friend whose husband of twenty-four years divorced her because he could not accept his wife's ileostomy.

"My first realization came, somewhat groggily, the first time the nurse emptied my post-op bag," she continued. "The doctor had not fully explained the surgery to me and I had no realization of what it would be like . . . reality came later when I got home and had to look at myself in a full-length mirror. I would have been better off with some prior knowledge, perhaps even some counseling."

We then asked what kind of nonverbal messages she got from the nursing staff.

> I remember that very clearly. I was taken care of by an older nurse and she was just wonderful. I was horrified when I saw the bag full of fecal matter and just apologized and apologized to her as I fought back tears of shame and embarrassment. She told me that it didn't bother her at all. I didn't believe her words but I sure did believe her behavior, because she took care of that bag just as nonchalantly as if she were washing her breakfast dishes. I think she is one of the reasons I decided to go into nursing. I got such excellent care, but I know that not all ileostomy patients do, and I was exposed to some of the other situations during my training.

> I saw patients receive insensitive care from nurses, and, if those patients knew as little in advance as I did, well, I just feel sorry for them, that's all. The nonverbal messages I got from that first nurse— messages that said you're okay—probably helped me more than anything else to adjust and go forward with my life. All the nurses who cared for me were compassionate. I was lucky! And, I know now that perceptive nurses know that emotional truth is expressed nonverbally.

> I sometimes saw nurses who really should go back to school. All they seemed to care about was getting the procedure done. They lacked compassion and made people feel . . . well, you just do it my way or I'm not going to take care of you. The poor patients lying there on their backs realized that they were not going to get care unless they performed the way the nurses wanted them to. As a student, I helped take care of an elderly colostomy patient who had cancer of the colon. She apologized to me for having to change the bag, just as I had done. The odor was bad, but I remembered the compassion showed me, talked gently to her and did the procedure as if it were as normal to me as doing my breakfast dishes. Sure, it took a little control. It does for everybody, but if the nurse can only think; 'There but for the grace of God, go I,' it will help. In my case, I had to think, there I was, and hope that I was able to help my patient as I had been helped.

CARDIAC PATIENTS

There is probably no area where it is more necessary to exercise a positive nonverbal behavioral attitude than in conjunction with the recovery and the rehabilitation of the cardiac patient. His rehabilitation is closely related to his emotional response to his illness. One of the primary functions of rehabilitation is helping the patient to develop a healthy mental attitude toward his condition and toward the future. To most patients, a heart attack means "dropping dead" or a life of semi-invalidism. This is obviously based more on popular fallacy than on fact, because a great number of cardiac patients return to normal living. However, the patient does need to understand the nature of his condition.

It is important for the cardiac patient to receive reinforcement. The failure of the physician to discuss prognosis and to help the patient plan for the future may create emotional anxiety and tensions that affect his recovery.

A person's attitude toward heart disease can have a very real effect on his chances for recovery. Some people are so frightened that they are almost afraid to move and give up every activity, while, in truth, all they need do is be more careful.

Some forms of heart disease can be cured, while others can be controlled and made bearable by treatment. The patient should have a good understanding of how a normal heart works. He should know what to do in the case of a subsequent attack. When a patient knows that certain things bring on an attack he can learn to be more careful behaviorally.

Myocardial Infarction (Coronary Occlusion)

Myocardial infarction is also referred to as MI, heart attack, or coronary thrombosis. Myocardial infarction is the sudden blocking of one or more of the coronary arteries. If it involves an extensive area, death results. If it is less extensive, it will result in necrosis of heart tissue and subsequent scarring. Other vessels can take over for the injured area if the scarring is not too extensive.

The myocardial attack begins suddenly with a sharp severe pain in the chest, sometimes radiating to the left arm and shoulder. It is similar to angina, but lasts longer and is more severe; exertion may have nothing to do with bringing on an attack. Also, unlike angina, it does not go away with rest, and nitroglycerin and amyl nitrite do not help.

Nonverbal signs that may be observed during a myocardial infarction are the patient's restlessness, the constant pacing around, and the ashen, cold, or clammy skin. He is dyspneic, cyanotic, and has a rapid, thready pulse; his blood pressure drops.

Nursing care is centered around these nonverbal signs and symptoms. Interpreting these nonverbal signs is vital to the patient's well-being, and so are the nursing measures. The patient can feel more secure, perhaps less restless, when he senses your consideration for his need for assistance in providing for his physical comfort.

The focus of treatment and care is to provide complete physical and mental quiet and rest. The patient needs to know that his light signal and any other item he needs or wants are within easy reach. Plan his care so that he has periods of rest and feels relaxed. Observe him for signs of fatigue. The observation and understanding of nonverbal signs relating to the patient's condition may not be thought of as communication, but it is this nonverbal language that the professional must understand while treating the cardiac patient.

Cerebral Vascular Accident

The cerebral vascular accident (CVA) is brought on by a sudden interruption of the blood supply to some vital center in the brain. It is known as apoplexy and often referred to as shock. It may be caused gradually by cerebral thrombosis, or suddenly by a cerebral embolism. It may cause complete or partial paralysis or death.

With a cerebral hemorrhage, the CVA happens suddenly with very little, if any, warning; sometimes, the patient feels dizzy or has a strange sensation in his head just before he collapses. He may become unconscious, his face is red, and he breathes noisily and with difficulty. His pulse is slow, but full and bounding. His blood pressure is elevated, and he may be in a deep coma, which becomes deeper and deeper until he dies, or he may gradually regain consciousness and eventually recover. Patients who are comatose for a long period of time are less likely to recover.

The patient who is not comatose may have a poor memory or inconsistent behavior; he may be easily fatigued, may lose bowel and bladder control, or have poor balance. Often, he is paralyzed on one side with loss of movement or sensation or both.

The most common result of a CVA is hemiplegia, or paralysis of one side of the body. It should be remembered that the nerves from one side of the brain cross over to the opposite side of the body; if the left side of the brain is injured, the right side of the body will be paralyzed or incapacitated in some way. The patient may not be able to see on one side, or he may see double. Other functions may also be impaired, such as hearing, general sensation, and circulation. It all depends on what part of the brain is affected. If the speech center of the brain is damaged, the result may be aphasia, which is the loss of the ability to use or to understand the spoken or the written language. Many patients recover some speech, but others never do.

MASTECTOMIES _____

The breast is the most common site of cancer in women. The prognosis for cure depends primarily on the extent of the disease at the time of treatment, as determined by the location and the size of the lesion, the presence or the absence of the axillary node involvement, and the number and the location of positive nodes. The best possible prognosis can be made when an early diagnosis is combined with the appropriate therapy. The nationwide movement to educate women about breast cancer, the techniques of breast self-examination, and the need for comprehensive breast examination are aimed at improving the rate, time, and quality of survival.

Primary breast cancer is usually treated by the surgical removal of the entire breast and of the axillary lymph nodes, with or without the removal of the pectoralis major muscle. The extent of surgery is determined by the size and the location of the lesion, the patient's age and general physical and emotional condition, and evidence of metastases. Radical mastectomy is based on the concept that wide excision of the overlying skin, the entire breast and the pectoralis major muscle, along with careful dissection of the axillary lymph nodes, will result in the removal of the primary tumor and its immediate sites of metastases. Frequently referred to as the classical radical mastectomy, it has been reported to yield a lower local recurrence rate and a higher ten-year survival rate than any other surgical method of treatment.

The nursing care of patients undergoing radical mastectomy for breast cancer is aimed at minimizing or preventing the physical complications and emotional strains associated with this surgery.

When a lump in her breast is discovered, a woman's emotional reactions are immediately set into motion. She is acutely aware that the lesion may be cancerous. Suddenly, she is faced with thoughts of mutilation and a life-threatening illness, and anxiety and denial begin to operate.

The patient's psychological rehabilitation begins with the initial nurse-patient contact. The nurse's willingness to take the time to listen, and her obvious concern will promote the patient's confidence and trust, both in the nurse and in the surgeon.

Most mastectomy patients arrive at the hospital full of dread and apprehension. Many, when interviewed, admitted that a great deal of their communication took place on a nonverbal level. Almost all postmastectomy patients are in constant fear of losing the remaining breast, and they often experience phantom pains and imagine tumors. Such subjective symptoms require a liberal dose of nursing reassurance and solicitude, a kind of medicine for despair. One young patient said that the worst part of her experience was going through two operations: the first with almost full assurance that the lesion was benign, and the second, knowing she had cancer.

Another forty-year-old patient said:

A smile and kindness are what help you get well. I communicated with my doctor and two nurses, in particular, nonverbally. I trusted them so much, and they were so compassionate. We just seemed to know what the other one thought.

She went on to say:

My two surgeries were nine days apart. I was sitting in the chair one day, after my first surgery, and Doctor J. came in. He sat down in front of me and cupped my face in his hands and he just looked at me. I knew without any words that I would have to have another surgery. I cried, and he just patted my face until I stopped crying.

Much later this same patient said, "I knew when the doctor walked into my room whether it was going to be a good day or not." Before she left the hospital, I heard this patient say, "Thank you, doctor, for saving my life, I've learned a lot from it, because now I know that I can do anything I have to do."

Another patient was able to tell that her student nurse had undergone the same kind of surgery. The student did not verbalize this and the patient said, "Somehow I just knew it. Without any words. It was her compassion and the way she touched me and cared for me. So, I asked her and she said 'Yes. I know how you feel and I want to help you.' " This patient went on to say, "I had the same nurse for the rest of my hospitalization, and every day was a good day after that."

For many women, feelings of self-esteem, desirability, and sexuality are closely related to the breast. The nurse who is gentle when she does a mastectomy dressing says nonverbally that her patient has dignity and self-esteem, that the cure of her operative area is personal and important and should be done with privacy, as if she had a breast. An understanding nurse knows that in our culture breasts have been idealized, have come to symbolize a woman's sexuality, and that the loss of one or both breasts can be a very traumatic experience.

The patient's ability to adapt to disfigurement depends not only on its extent, but also on how she emotionally experiences it. This, in turn, is related to her body image and to her previously existing personality. The nature of her emotional and perceptual reaction will also vary over the course of time. A compassionate nurse knows that anxiety reaction is related to fear of rejection by others because of the disfigurement and because the abruptness of the alteration in body appearance has not yet permitted the formation of a new body image. Patients with disfigurement also react with depression, since any alteration in the body image is experienced as a loss of a body part and as a reduction of self-esteem. These are additional reasons why it is important for the nurse to accept the disfigurement and enable the patient to feel accepted as a whole person. Once again, gentleness with the mastectomy dressing serves as an ideal way to nonverbally convey acceptance of the patient and of her disfigurement. Another way the nurse can accomplish this is to look directly at the operative site and not show any signs of withdrawal.

LIMB AMPUTATIONS

Although the concept of loss is generally discussed in relation to dying and to death, there are patients who have experienced other kinds of significant losses. With modern advances in medical treatment and surgical techniques, limb amputations have become prevalent. A total of 35,000 limb amputations are performed in the United States annually.

Limb amputations are most often a result of highway accidents, and they happen to people of all ages. The body and body parts may be conceived of as good or bad, pleasing or repulsive, clean or dirty, loved or disliked. Such attitudes and values about the body are an integral part of the body image.

The phantom limb, for example, is an almost universal reaction following amputation, and reflects an aspect of the body image that is anchored in a neurophysiological substrate developed fairly early in life. The phantom phenomenon is observed after removal of a body part such as a breast, penis, nose, nipple, and, certainly, most commonly after amputation of limbs. Generally, the greater movement of a body part, the more sharply defined will be a later phantom. Most amputees will report some physical sensation associated with the lost extremity. Immediately following amputation, the patient usually experiences the phantom as the entire extremity, the distal portion most vividly. The sensations may be tingling "pins and needles," or disagreeably painful sensations. The initial experience of the phantom gradually diminishes for most patients. With some patients, the total disappearance of the phenomenon may take as long as several years. It is of interest to note that children who have amputations before the age of six or seven, or children who are born without limbs, do not experience the phantom phenomenon, reflecting the fact that the neurophysiological patterns of body image are not firmly established before this time. It is important for the nurse who is communicating therapeutically to acknowledge that psychogenic pain in the stump or the phantom pain does exist, and that it is real for the patient. The expression on the nurse's face can convey her feelings and will either deny or confirm that she believes the pain is real. Prolonged and unremitting phantom pain is considered to be pathological.

There are many discouraging moments for the patient with an artificial leg or prosthesis as he fights to overcome awkwardness and embarrassment. Free and open communication with the nurse can go a long way toward encouraging these patients.

Adaptation is the process of change and the reestablishment of a steady state. When it occurs, the patient is able to retain his integrity and his sense of wholeness within the reaction of his environment. Real adaptation must include the response to environmental change. After the physiological insult has occurred, the patient has one of three choices. First, the patient can adapt by reaching a dependent steady state, one in which he never moves beyond the limits of his illness. An example of this is the cardiac patient who reaches a state of dependency and decides to spend the rest of his life in bed or the spinal injury patient who depends on others to meet his needs and to perform his previous duties.

Second, the patient may react by denying that a physiological crisis has occurred. In this category would be patients with emphysema who continue to smoke; the patient with a perforated ulcer who believes that antacids will cure his problem, as he continues an intense and pressured work pace; the MI patient who feels that his condition is due to lack of rest and who counts on two weeks in the hospital for a cure. Such behavior may be hazardous, but rather than face certain limitations in his activity, the patient ignores the severity of the entire experience.

The third choice is positive adaptation. The patient can choose to establish a new steady state, in which he realistically integrates the past crisis and the future limitations into a new life. This patient has learned from his illness experience. It is essential that the nurse interpret the course of action the patient has chosen. It is axiomatic that if the nurse understands the patient's problem, she will cooperate in reinforcing the behaviors that lead to positive adaptation. If the nurse determines that the patient has made the right choice, she should not paternalize, but should accept him as the whole person he was before. It is up to the nurse to identify negative adaptation and to help the patient to adapt more positively. The nurse must formulate a plan of action based upon open communication: she should encourage the patient to communicate his fears, frustrations, and anxieties about the future. She can pick up many nonverbal cues from his face and actions. The nurse can help him to develop a new future based upon assessment of the past and appraisal of realistic goals or limitations. Ideally, her support and understanding will enable the patient to accept any limitations.

The patient needs continual positive reinforcement (touch, a smile at the right time) in order to adapt positively. He must realize that, regardless of what brought him into the present experience and situation, he does have future value. By becoming aware of his value to others, he becomes more hopeful of the future. Ideally he looks forward to going home and getting his life back in order. The patient who positively adapts should realize that adaptation will continue in an even broader sense once he is home.

4
Pediatrics and Mothering

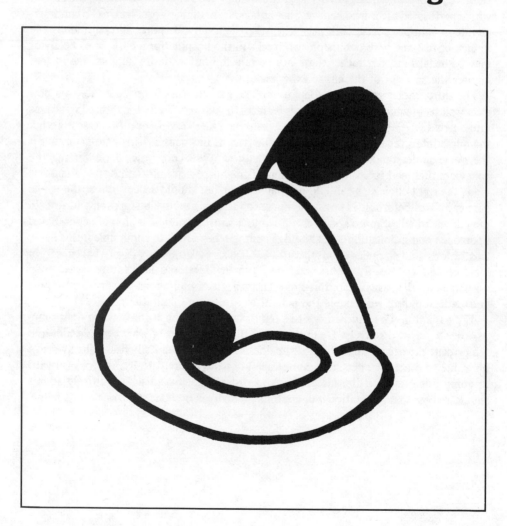

It is interesting that we have to relearn nonverbal communication as adults, since we were able to understand it long before we were able to respond to verbal symbols. Nonverbal communication begins at birth when the newborn baby's first cry brings comfort to the mother and the baby, in turn, is comforted by the warmth of his mother's body. We react nonverbally before we understand words. Obviously, there is very little verbal comprehension or expression early in life. However, this verbal void does not preclude an interpretation of such nonverbal cues as touch. As an infant matures, he begins to understand what the parent figure is attempting to convey through a combination of verbal and nonverbal actions. During this early stage of growth, he begins to interpret first nonverbal behavior, then a combination of verbal and nonverbal symbols, and, finally, words.

The infant is comforted by the feel of the nipple in his mouth. Later, he will come to recognize a bottle as a symbol, that which satisfies his hunger, and will stop fussing when he sees it in his mother's hand. Feeding is usually accompanied by words. The mother says "here's baby's bottle; it's time for baby's bottle." The child will eventually attempt to imitate his mother's sounds. The first attempts may come out sounding more like "baba," but with maturation he will master the sound.

His infantile, exclusively nonverbal behavior will be modified as his proficiency with words develops. A five-year-old, for example, can be quite articulate when asking for a bottle of soda pop. Under stress, young children frequently revert to earlier behavior patterns. This is observable in the pediatrics ward when the six-year-old, with an adequate vocabulary, suddenly begins to point toward the desired object, cry, or use baby talk. The child has not lost his verbal ability. He is merely reacting to the stress of pain or fright by regressing into an infantile behavioral pattern.

Perception is acute in the preverbal child. Although he himself cannot talk or understand the speech of others, he senses many things that go on around him. Without understanding the cause, he will feel and react to fear, anger, or sadness, just as surely as he will react to a wet diaper or a hungry stomach. Therefore, the loving care an infant receives is just as important as his physical care. The gentle care of the baby is a nonverbal expression of love. It contributes to his feeling of security and makes such physical care as bathing and feeding pleasurable. Infants should be given as much touch contact as possible: holding, hugging, fondling, rocking. Studies show that twenty minutes of extra handling will result in earlier exploring and grasping behavior. Therefore, the nursing staff, who are surrogate mothers during the baby's hospitalization, should take every opportunity to hold and to touch the babies. This nonverbal communication of love and security is necessary for the baby's physical and mental development.

After any painful procedure, the nurse should hold the baby lovingly for a few minutes, so that he does not associate only pain with her care. Murmuring, which is a nonverbal behavior, and talking softly will further enhance the baby's sense of trust.

The infant is sensitive to touch. Touch provides the first impressions of life—security, warmth, love, and pleasure. Through touch, the infant gains his first knowledge of the people around him. The physician, delivery room nurse, nursery nurse, and the mother are the first to touch the newborn. The infant soon learns to recognize his mother's touch, and to feel and react to her sense of anxiety, lack of confidence, anger, or rejection. Early touch experiences and the infant's perceptions through them apparently lay the foundation for his feelings for people throughout life.

Visceral sensations of discomfort, hunger, overdistention of the stomach, passage of gas in the stool, and extremes of temperature account for much of the newborn's crying. At first, his cry is simply a primitive discharge mechanism, a call for help. Crying brings comfort from the mother. In a few weeks, the baby acquires subtle modifications in the sound of his cry; these give the mother cues about the nature of his discomfort. She begins to recognize the hungry cry, the wet cry, and to adjust her response to fit the baby's needs.

The birth cry, the result of reflex action, is considered to be the first speech uttered, the most primitive process of phonation. Other early vocalizations consist of cooing and babbling. At this time, the baby should hear sounds from adults and children around him, as he will begin to imitate those sounds. To do this he moves his tongue with vocalization; this process is called lalling. The first sound is "ammm" when crying. At this time, the infant begins to vocalize wordless recognition of people. His sounds begin to mean certain objects. He begins to understand words that indicate scolding or praise. He may cry at the sound of "no" and smile at "pretty baby."

This imitative stage is different from the spontaneous, early babbling. It is a form of vocal play with the added pleasure of imitation. Before true speech, he invents sounds for objects. "La" may mean food, toy, or light. During this stage, the infant's language is autistic; he associates meaning with his own sounds, but those sounds are unintelligible to other people. Most of the sounds of infancy are universal.

The developmental crisis for infancy is trust versus mistrust (Erikson, Erik. *Childhood and Society.*)[10] Basic trust involves confidence, optimism, reliance on self and others, faith that the world can satisfy needs, and a sense of hope or belief in the attainability of wishes in spite of problems.

Mistrust is a sense of not feeling satisfied emotionally or physically. It is characterized by pessimism, lack of self-confidence, suspicion and bitterness toward others, and antagonism. A person feels that things just will not turn out right. The nurse should tell the new mother that security and trust are fostered by prompt, skillful, consistent response to the infant's distress and needs, as well as by positive response to his happy behavior. The cry is a distress signal, and the parents do not spoil a baby by promptly answering his cry. Instead, they are teaching trust by relieving his tension.

The nurse should help the parents to understand the meaning they convey through such care as changing diapers. The baby will sense a positive attitude if one exists. If the parents constantly fail to meet his primary needs, then fear, anger, insecurity and, eventually, mistrust result. If and when the most important people fail him, he has little foundation on which to build trust and faith in others or in himself. Later, he will have trouble socializing. He will feel the world cannot be trusted. Trust is developed on a nonverbal level, and touch contacts are especially necessary to create trust.

Parent–child communication begins at birth; therefore, natural childbirth may offer some additional benefits to parents. The mother can feel secure on a minimum of anesthetics and analgesics and because she is awake she can participate in the delivery. She can see and touch her baby immediately after the birth, and a mutual bond is developed.

Today, many fathers are included as more and more young couples try to share in childbirth. Both parents can attend prenatal classes and learn the signs and the sensations that are to be expected. The husband can support his wife throughout the entire birth process.

The baby benefits from prepared childbirth. He will be more alert and responsive, for he will not be subject to the depressant effect of narcotics received by the mother.

When the mother first holds her baby after delivery a closeness is felt. When this occurs, a stage has been successfully set for the development of trust; yet, not one word has been spoken. The entire communication took place with touch and holding, looking, and feeling.

One of the major causes of failure to thrive in newborns is maternal deprivation; prepared childbirth can prevent this. Maternal deprivation may also occur when a previously warm relationship with the mother is interrupted in the second six months. Perceptual deprivation—lack of tactile, vestibular, visual, or auditory stimuli—is another cause for failure to thrive. Mothering is a form of communication, and it is an essential component to the well-being of the newborn child. When the infant is hospitalized, the nursing staff either share in the mothering role or become surrogate mothers.

French obstetrician Frederick Le Boyer[11] states that the standard delivery room practices of the past create a birth trauma in infants. He believes that the baby's birth should be a gentle transition from womb to world. In order to accomplish this smooth transition, the delivery room should be kept dim and quiet. This prevents the baby from being confronted with bright operating room lamps and loud noises. The newborn is never held upside down by his feet, but handled gently. In this way, the spine is not jerked from its fetal position. As the infant emerges from the uterus, he is carefully placed on his mother's abdomen with the umbilical cord still uncut. Then the baby is gently massaged, and his limbs slowly unfold. When the newborn is no longer receiving oxygen from the mother's placenta, the umbilical cord is cut, and the baby is immersed in comforting lukewarm water. This first bath closely resembles the environment of the uterus from which the baby has so recently departed.

Dr. Le Boyer feels that this method of entering the world creates natural sleeping patterns, that it fosters a healthy psyche in the newborn, which will permit him to thrive in his new environment. This method is seen by many as a soothing, nonverbal entry into the world.

In caring for infants, pediatric nurses fill a dual role. They care for the baby's physical and medical needs, and they also fill his need for mothering. If the mothering needs are not met in early infancy, the baby may fail to grow and to develop physically and emotionally. The most important nonverbal tool in nursing infants is touch.

PREMATURE INFANTS

The gestation period in humans is ten lunar months, or 280 days. Babies born before forty weeks are considered to be premature. They are physically immature and run increased risks of illness and death. The normal gestation period is also known as nine calendar months, or term.

Babies born before term present special care problems. They should not be subjected to unnecessary exposure or to the dangers of trauma and infection. At first, the cardinal rules are to handle the "preemie" as little as possible, to minimize sensory stimulation. The preemie has been inadvertently removed from the normal and friendly environment of the mother's protective womb into the hostile outside world before term. There is a need to accommodate the special needs of the baby to compensate for the period of development and maturation that would have been supplied by the mother and her placenta if the baby had remained in the uterus until term.

The nursery and its special equipment provide the baby with an environment similar in many ways to the friendly environment of the mother's uterus and acts as a surrogate parent during the period of adjustment to the outside world. Health professionals, who have watched preemies grow, believe that there is a higher incidence among them of poor growth, lower intelligence, unwillingness to socialize, parental rejection, and child abuse. It suggests that these problems stem from the preemie's early sensory deprivation and separation from the parents. As a result, it is recognized by many professionals that the baby has a need to touch the mother's face, as well as to hear her voice from the earliest possible moment. Involvement of the parents in as many ways as possible, after the initial crisis of premature birth has passed and the baby is admitted to the intensive care nursery, is recommended. The parents should be allowed to touch their child. This first touch is the beginning of nonverbal communication between them. The parents should be allowed to touch the baby even if the infant is critically ill. Then, if the infant dies, the parents will be more able to cope with their grief and do so without unnecessary guilt feelings.

It is of special interest to the parents to be able to see and to handle the baby during the feeding. If the baby is on nasogastric feeding, parents can touch and hold their baby through the Isolette portholes while the nurse administers the feeding. If the baby's temperature is stable and he can be taken out of the Isolette for a short while, wrapped in blankets, the mother or father can hold, rock, or talk to him while he is being fed. Although talking is normally considered a form of verbal communication, at this level of the infants comprehension, it is considered to be nonverbal.

The handling of the baby by the parents during the time he is confined to the Isolette promotes a more natural transition for the time when the parents can provide the necessary care for his well-being at home. The same intimate nonverbal practice of touching the child, accompanied by soft cooing and chatter, should be continued and increased in the baby's new at-home environment. This tends to assure the healthy development of the child. Once the premature infant has gained the status of the healthy full-term baby, he has an excellent chance of becoming a healthy adult, and he may very well live as long as other adults.

TODDLERS

Each child is an individual. Just as no two babies look alike, no two are the same in disposition and activity. This becomes more evident as children reach the toddler stage. Toddlers present a communication problem in pediatric care because there is no standard vocabulary level. One four-year-old child may be quite articulate, while another is very limited. In dealing with young children, the nurse is on safe ground when she uses all her nonverbal techniques. Facial expression is important; children look to adult facial expressions for signs of approval or disapproval. A smile goes a long way in establishing rapport with a small child. Touch contacts reassure him—being warm and friendly, giving a pat on the head, hand, or arm lets him know that he is in safe territory.

Young children are often afraid, but this is not the same fear older patients experience. Nurses become acquainted with adult fear, which is based on the reality of a poor prognosis or impending surgery. Small children are too young to understand life, death, and serious illness in adult terms. They are afraid because they are in an unfamiliar setting, surrounded by strange faces, and they feel that they have been deserted by their parents. The fear is increased by pain and discomfort.

Environment is important in pediatric areas. Most hospitals recognize this and design the pediatric units to be as comfortable, colorful, and unhospital-like as possible. Toys, dolls, and stuffed animals are available for the children, and some youngsters will insist on bringing a favorite toy or stuffed animal with them to the hospital. The toy from home will be very important to the child and should not be taken from him unless absolutely necessary.

The toddler can be made more comfortable by careful observation of his behavioral cues— what makes him cry? What quiets him? What makes him smile? The younger the child, the more the need for touching. Some children are suddenly absent from their parents for the first time in their lives. They are frightened and miss mothering. If they are accustomed to being nursed or rocked, they will be deprived when the comfort contact is taken away without offering some substitute. Holding and rocking are excellent techniques. With children up to about the age of four, there is no substitute for touch contacts.

PLAY THERAPY

Young children spend their time in play. Play is a natural activity. Recent investigations stress the importance of play to the sick child's physical, mental, emotional, and social development. A child's play helps him to develop coordination of muscles and exercises all parts of his body. He uses up energy, develops self-confidence, communicates with other children, and advances another step in his development. There are many forms of play. Some will help the child learn colors, sizes, shapes, and textures; others will help him develop motor skills and muscle coordination. The child's enthusiasm for play should be tapped by the nurse, since it provides a good opportunity for her to come into close contact with him. The nurse will learn a great deal about her young patient as she observes him at play.

Play experience is usually included in the student nurse's training period. To be of assistance, the nurse must understand the needs of the child. She can accomplish this by picking up the numerous nonverbal cues sent by the youngster. Sometimes, a student will take refuge in some activity that takes her away from the child, i.e., at the desk after the morning cares are done, reading the patient's chart for too long a time. This may indicate that she feels insecure and inadequate with the child after his physical care is completed. She may feel sorry for the child, but she does not know what to do for him, so she frequently finds herself busy elsewhere. If she has learned the needs of a child and the value of play therapy, she will not need to feel guilty; she does not withdraw from the child any longer. The pediatric experience then becomes fulfilling and rewarding for her. The child who carefully and calmly builds a house of blocks may be suggesting, nonverbally, that he is at peace. The child who roughly bangs and pounds or throws the blocks may nonverbally be suggesting he is angry or restless or anxious.

In providing suitable play for children of various ages in the hospital, there are a number of factors to be considered. The patient's state of health has to be considered. This will determine the amount of activity in which he can participate. The nurse can provide many activities that will relieve stress and provide enjoyment for the patient on bedrest. Overstimulation would be hazardous for the severely ill child, e.g., the child with a cardiac diagnosis, who needs to conserve his strength. The nurse should always be on guard for signs of fatigue in her patient and act accordingly.

The nurse should know what toys should be safe, durable, and suited to the child's developmental level. Of course, toys should not be sharp, nor should they have parts that are easily removed and swallowed. Too many toys at one time are confusing to the child, just as complicated toys are frustrating. Well-selected toys such as balls, blocks, dolls, have been useful throughout the years. Each child should be given sufficient time to complete the activity. Usually, quiet play should precede meals and bedtime. Boys and girls seem to enjoy similar toys. Sometimes, it will be necessary to take a youngster by the hand and lead him into activities with other children.

Many activities are performed and observed nonverbally, e.g., finger play, scrapbooks, collections of scrap material containing bright ribbons, bits of string, old popsicle sticks, coat hangers, pipe cleaners, paper bags, newspapers. Some other nonverbal communication can be provided by the radio, phonograph, and piano. Drawings, finger paints, and modeling clay foster creativity. The latter merely require a flat surface, such as the overbed table and the particular medium. The use of rubber sheets to protect the bed permits the child on bedrest to participate in messy projects. The child confined to a crib can participate if his back is supported by pillows or by elevating the mattress.

The nurse can help her pediatric patient develop socially. To do this she must acquire knowledge about the stages of growth and development; for instance, the one-year-old can play near other children, while the two-year-old pushes and grabs. The latter has his own way of acknowledging other children. The preschool child is getting ready for cooperative play. The ability to socialize increases during the school years.

SCHOOL-AGE CHILDREN

As children grow older they begin to realize what serious illness and death mean in adult terms. Lois Jean Davitz in *Interpersonal Process in Nursing: Case Histories*[12] writes of a nine-year-old who was born with multiple heart defects. The pediatrics unit had become a familiar world to the youngster. The treatment, mainly heart stimulants, diuretics, and oxygen were neither painful nor unpleasant, and the young patient enjoyed her stay, referring to the hospital as her second home. But on her final admission, the usually talkative, smiling child was silent and unresponsive. One of the staff nurses had been present at the patient's birth and involved with her care on each subsequent admission. This nurse was a great favorite of the youngster's. One day the patient asked, "Am I pretty?" The nurse replied that she was indeed very pretty. The youngster then said, "Will I be pretty when I grow up?" The nurse responded by saying, "I'll just pull the sheet up here." The youngster became pale and refused to speak for the rest of the day. The child was extremely bright and had begun to realize the seriousness of her own condition, even to fear death, a fear that was confirmed by her interpretation of the nurse's verbal and nonverbal response.

Children with serious health problems, such as congenital defects, face multiple hospitalizations during their childhood. They may, as the youngster cited above, change drastically in their response to those hospitalizations as they grow older— perhaps because they have grown old enough to realize the seriousness of their own poor prognosis, or merely because they are going through a growing-up procedure compounded by the additional problem of congenital or long-term illness or disability.

The school-age youngster will not want to be treated like a baby. And he will resent or dislike the doctor or nurse who treats him so. Procedures can be explained to him and phrased in a way that he will understand. The child should be told the truth about a procedure that will hurt. Some people in nursing will still respond to the child's question "will it hurt?" by saying "no," when they know that it will hurt. When this happens the child will not trust the nurse to tell him the truth the next time he has a question. He may even distrust all nurses. It is better for the nurse to say, "Yes, this will hurt, but just for a moment, and then when it's over with, the pain in your head, or the pain in your arm will be gone, too."

Children do not like grouchy nurses. A six-year-old, in speaking of his hospitalization, said, "If I were a nurse, I would be nice to people. I'd be nice to people and not have a grouchy face. And I wouldn't tell children lies either, saying something wouldn't hurt when it did."

In the elementary school years, girls generally prefer to play with girls and boys with boys. Children can play in playrooms or in the wards. The type of illness each child has must be considered for his own protection. Sometimes, it is helpful for a child to play with younger children, for this offers him release from competition with his peers. On the other hand, too much play with younger children may tend to make him fall behind his peer group in physical skills and in language abilities. Also, sometimes older children tend to dominate. This can lead to bickering and to disruption of play with the younger children. The nurse, therefore, must learn to set limits. She can convey authority without anger or threat. She must be positive, clear, and consistent so the child will know what is acceptable behavior. When the occasion arises, she will place specific limits on special actions. At the same time, she must maintain some flexibility in rules. This is not always easy and requires time and patience. As the nurse learns to recognize the child's wish, and when that wish is not permissible, she may say: "You wish you could do that, but . . ." When restrictions are imposed, children often express or act out of resentment. When this happens, the rules should be stated kindly but firmly.

Some pediatric patients must be isolated because of medical necessities, such as communicable disease, burns, requirements for total rest, and traction. The pediatrics nurse will be challenged to find appropriate stimulation and socialization for such children, and she may have to provide some of the socialization or arrange for it through outsiders or hospital volunteers.

Preadolescent children are often less talkative than older and younger children, and they withdraw when frustrated, instead of verbalizing their hostility. A healthy outlet for these children is to let them share their feelings with their best friend, and that friend many times is their nurse, who can listen, converse, and help the youngster work through his problems. Children understand language directed at their feelings; this is another reason why nonverbal communication used with them is so useful.

A therapeutic nurse should have a philosophy that encourages a child toward maturity. She will have to have a sense of humor and be fair, considerate, and friendly. Being familiar with child development will also enable her to recognize the different stages of growth and development that each child goes through. When young patients become problems, it is probably because they have problems. A good approach is to sit down and talk with them. You can say: "I know you're worried. Do you want to talk about it?" If they can begin talking about it, their feelings come out, and the problem behavior usually subsides.

HANDICAPPED CHILDREN

Handicapped children also provide a challenge. A blind or a deaf child may not be able to relate to a peer group in play or in the wards, at least not the same as a child with normal vision or hearing. Mentally retarded children require more stimulation and a realization that the child's chronological and mental age are not the same. For example, an eight-year-old mentally retarded youngster may be more comfortable playing with the younger children than he would be with his own group. And indeed, his capabilities mentally would be more in line with that of the younger children.

The hospitalized child who will spend many months or years in a facility is considered to have a long-term chronic illness. He may be physically or mentally handicapped. Such a child may occasionally be taken out to movies, the circus, or restaurants, so that he can learn about the outside world. They often have language disorders, and they tend to use nonverbal communication much more than other children. Special accommodations are improvised for these children. One example, when they have to remain on their backs, would be mirrors for reading. Electrical page-turners are also handy for the handicapped. Cassette tapes are often used for the quadriplegics so they can enjoy and derive some human pleasure from being involved.

Some of the types of handicaps are a result of cerebral palsy, juvenile arthritis, heart disorders, and orthopedic impairment. These are but a few of the congenital anomalies that require limited physical activity. These children can derive a great deal of pleasure from watching television, especially when it is adapted to their age level and comprehension, and from listening to records, stories, and music.

On occasion, these children need to be admitted to an acute hospital facility. When this happens, it is usually an emotional upset for the child, since the significant others in his life have suddenly been changed. The facility they just came from was home, and the nurses there were surrogate mothers. What a challenge for the acute facility nurse who cares for such a youngster.

In this crisis there will be a great deal of nonverbal communication, for often there is fear on the child's face and a sense of awkwardness in the nurse. Each is a stranger. And each is expressing his feelings without words.

SPECIAL BEHAVIORS

Destructive behavior such as head banging is often observed in disturbed or retarded children. However, not all destructive behavior is abnormal. For some children, head banging is a normal developmental phenomenon. Nonpathological head banging begins in the second six months of life and may persist for about seventeen months. When it continues beyond the age of four, or becomes so frequent or severe that it causes injury, it is considered abnormal. The traditional nursing approach to this behavior is to restrain the child. While restraints offer physical protection to the child, they do limit his freedom. Perhaps a better approach would be to interpret the behavior as much as possible and then try to develop and to reinforce more positive behaviors. To do this, it is important to have good nursing observation. When does the behavior occur? How many times a day? What other things are happening when the behavior occurs? What causes it? When observations produce these data, the nursing staff can then intervene to develop substitute activities or perhaps just sit and hold or rock the child during the time when he is most inclined to bang his head.

Hospitalization can be traumatic to anyone. It is especially so to children. Therefore, it is a very good idea if the child can be given a tour of the hospital before his admission. Let him handle and become familiar with some of the equipment that he will use. These techniques will decrease his fear of the unknown. He will be more able to cooperate in his treatment plan. Some hospitals have even instituted a program in which student nurses visit the families at home before the scheduled admission. The program was planned not only to help the children but also to help the nursing students realize what hospitalization means for a young child. The student nurse gathers all the available data before visiting the child. She then promises to see him again when he is in the hospital, and she does.

ADOLESCENCE

The adolescent has an identity conflict increased by his developing sexuality. Many nurses see him as too old for pediatrics, and many nurses on the other wards see him as too young for the adult wards.

The adolescent personality is frustrating to others and confusing to the youngster himself. Most adolescents have an overexaggerated concern with themselves. They want to be heard and noticed, but often turn shy and confused when they are. They are developing their values systems, want accurate information, and quickly lose trust in any adult who lies to them. If the adolescent youngster is going to have anesthesia, explain what it means: that he will feel nothing, and that he will not wake up during the surgery. Continue to tell him that he may have some pain after the surgery, but that there will be available medication to control it.

The adolescent may not totally understand your explanation, so repeat when necessary. Adolescents are frequently accused of being rebellious and of having disruptive behavior when, in actuality, their behavior is only a result of frustration because of the inadequate responses of adults.

Most adolescents do not like to be bossed, and it is a wise nurse who recognizes this and who involves the youngster in his own care plan whenever possible. Let him, when possible, decide when to have a bath, or the time a certain procedure should be done, or choose between one of several activities. When he has some voice in his own care, he is more likely to accept it, and to relate better to the nursing staff.

As secondary sexual characteristics develop, the adolescent has feelings about sex and about his own body. He may become shy about the bodily functions, and hospitals are not always the best places for privacy. The nurse, however, can help by using screens, especially when treatment of a personal nature is given, and by trying to see that the youngster is not walked in on while showering or using the bedpan.

Adolescents sometimes develop crushes on doctors or nurses and go through the whole giggling, blushing, love-note writing procedure. When this happens to you, you must be very careful not to belittle the youngster, or to laugh, no matter how comic the circumstances. You must not, of course, flirt back. A friendly, " you're okay, I'm okay" attitude works the best.

Adolescents need activity, and the TV alone will not suffice to meet this need. If your adolescent patient is restricted to bed, you will have to use a great deal of ingenuity to think up activities. Sometimes he will enjoy helping you with younger patients, but do not assume that he will.

When an adolescent patient is maimed or disfigured, he has problems with body image. A teenager who has had an amputation, for example, will probably not be comforted by your telling him that everything is going to work out. A better approach might be to say something like, "You're probably wondering what your friends at school are going to think, aren't you?" And then carry the conversation from there. An important part of effective nursing is not only to help repair the physical damage, but to help the patient face life after he leaves the hospital.

Adolescents often have dilemmas. They have to make choices for which they sometimes are not prepared or have not matured enough to make. When they cannot handle the dilemma, it can lead to illness. They may resent authority and guidance; they may feel hostile. The adolescent may have a need to be dependent and at the same time a desire to be independent. This is common to all adolescents. The nurse needs to be aware that the adolescent needs to work through his feelings of ambivalence and that this may often happen when he is hospitalized. Here the nurse can help him grow toward psychological maturity and to feel more secure. But to do this, she must be fair and objective. She can show concern and love, but she also has to set limits and not be overly permissive.

The nurse can learn a great deal about her adolescent patient by observing him and by actively listening to his views, and then she can determine how much freedom her patient can tolerate. The hospital environment should be as accepting and as emotionally stable as possible. Adolescence is yet another stage of growth and development where nonverbal communication is meaningful and useful. The adolescent patient is usually sensitive and perceptive. He does a great deal of quiet observation as he watches the nurses come and go, and he relates to this. The sensitive, perceptive nurse will join this patient in a warm and friendly manner. She will find these quiet times lead to better acceptance and to understanding between her and the patient. Both the nurse and the patient will learn how very much can be said without words and how good it can be.

In a mature environment, the mood swings of an adolescent need not baffle the nurse. The empathetic nurse is always aware of her adolescent patient's constant need in striving for self-esteem. She will accept her patient despite his human frailities, and when her young patient responds with warmth, friendliness, and appreciation she will realize that he is developing a healthy amount of self-esteem.

The nurse who opts to work in pediatrics should possess emotional maturity. She should have a good grip on her own emotions. She should be able to demonstrate a basic love for all children. Of course, no one can love everybody equally, but the nurse must be warm and accepting of all the children and their individual behavior patterns. Nurses who have young children of their own may find pediatrics difficult. They might relate too closely and find it just too hard to handle, especially when their relationship with the child is terminated. Pediatric nurses need the maturity to begin, to maintain, and to terminate relationships effectively.

5

Geriatrics

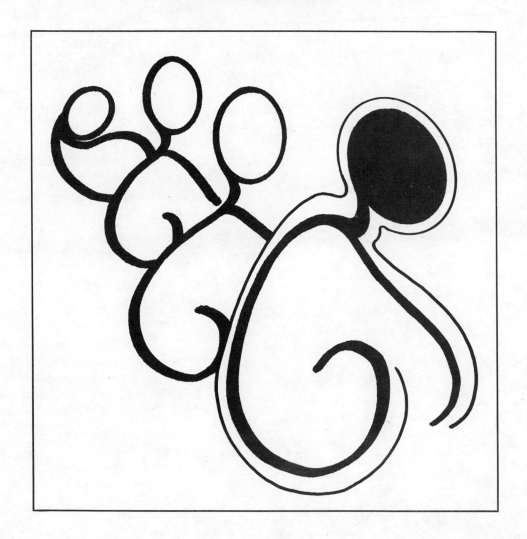

For most of us old age is a time of loss. Just as the worst of our struggles with the job and the family raising are behind, old age begins. Some visual acuity may be lost; some of us are wearing glasses by the time we are forty. With aging, hearing diminishes, and skin elasticity and muscle tone decrease; cancer, heart disease, and stroke take a mighty toll as the years pass. There are also environmental losses due to retirement and to professional obsolescence—standard of living is lowered with loss of income; children grow up and away; and friends and family members are lost to death. The fate of those we euphemistically label "senior citizens" was expressed poetically by Oliver Wendel Holmes:

And, if I should live to be
The last leaf upon the tree
In the Spring, let them smile
As I do now
At the old forsaken bough
Where I cling. (The Last Leaf)

With loss comes the sense of not belonging, problems with self-esteem, identity, and these feelings often bring about the greatest loss of all—loss of desire to continue living.

Because of these factors and others which will be covered later in this section, the geriatric nurse deals with people who are suffering deprivation in addition to illness. The emotional, social, and psychological needs of these patients must be considered in the delivery of skilled nursing care.

The geriatric situation is further complicated because rehabilitation cannot be measured by the same yardstick that we use in medical–surgical nursing. In fact, for many years, care of the elderly did not focus on rehabilitation. It was thought that the primary concern should be custodial care. This philosophy probably grew out of the fact that, in past years, old people without families or adequate funds were cared for custodially in charitable institutions, while their more solvent peers were looked after by family members or were able to hire a professional to deliver the needed care. The picture is quite different today. Modern geriatric care includes the rich and the poor, as well as older people who need complete nursing care, and a great number of people beyond retirement age whose needs can no longer be met by our society. Therefore, we can no longer be satisfied to meet only the basic need for food and shelter. We must, instead, attempt to restore each individual to the fullest level of health, ability, and happiness. The full measure of such rehabilitation can be accomplished if we learn to deal with the older patient's realities.

The need to deal with this problem is great, and it is immediate. Life expectancy for the average American has increased to 71 years. Twenty-two million Americans are already over the age of 65 (10% of our population); over the next decade this figure will undoubtedly double. Some forecasters predict that, by 1985, there will be more people over 65 than under 25.

Improved immunization, disease control, chemotherapy, and surgical procedures have contributed to this phenomenal shift in population age. Unfortunately, the cure and the control of the diseases of old age have not kept up with our rapidly expanding ability to keep people alive, so we face the social and the personal dilemma of increased life expectancy and decreased quality of life.

The increased numbers in the older population has created something of a power block. We read of "gray power" and the "senior" vote. This not-so-senile voice has been heard, and the national spotlight has been turned on the plight of the elderly. Governmental and social groups are dealing with their problems, especially in the areas of adequate housing and medical care.

In medical care of the aged, the geriatric nurse is the key person. When the "over-sixty-five" patient needs health attention, whether in an acute, extended care, skilled nursing, or restorative home health setting, the nurse is the primary person. Nursing has a special contribution to make to long-term and restorative care, and it is through nursing, more than anything else, that we can improve the quality of a person's last years. We will examine each of the geriatric environments later in this section, but, first, it is important to define the role of the geriatric nurse and to examine the qualities she needs, methods of delivery for her professional skills, and, especially, the dynamics of nonverbal communication in the geriatric setting.

GERIATRIC NURSING

Many nurses do not like geriatrics. It is not the most popular choice for newly graduated' nurses, with only a handful opting to work in this area, compared to the legions who seek assignments in medical–surgical, obstetrics, cardiac, and pediatric units. Yet, today's reality is that more and more nurses will be going into geriatrics because, as the older population increases, that is where the jobs will be.

Geriatrics has some negative connotations. We associate it with second-rate hospitals or homes for the old that just happen to have a nurse or two on staff. We think, mistakenly, of the long-term facility as a place for semiskilled nursing personnel or professional nurses who could not make it any place else. We look to the acute facility for our own careers. When we think this way, perhaps we are viewing the situation with too much pessimism and are seeing what was and too frequently still is, but which cannot and must not continue to be.

Geriatrics is taught in most nursing curricula, but often not given as much attention as other subject areas; therefore, many nurses do not understand it and are basically unprepared to cope with the multiple problems of the geriatric patient.

To be effective in geriatrics, nurses must be able to deliver skilled nursing care. This must come first, because without it all the lovely facilities and well-planned activities would be superfluous. Nurses must understand the diseases of old age, the meaning of chronicity, the importance of physical environment and space, the meaning of immobility, feelings of usefulness, and the patient's personal sense of impending death.

When nurses are aware and when they empathize with these special problems, they can plan skilled nursing care in meaningful terms. Just as with rehabilitation, geriatric care may have to be measured by a different yardstick.

The body system changes with age. Difficulties with digestion occur, circulation becomes poor, metabolism is slower, hearing and vision are decreased, the skin wrinkles, and people become easily chilled and less able to fight infections. These problems are sometimes exacerbated by more dramatic debilitation caused by diabetes, arthritis, rheumatism, sclerosis, and cardiac infarction.

The geriatric patient will need partial or continuous skilled nursing care to cope with any one or any combination of physical problems, but his needs will not end there. The effective nurse must recognize the older patient's other needs, which are social, environmental, and psychological, not really so different from the needs of other age groups. Whether we are 9 or 109, we all want to feel loved and valued for ourselves. But with the passing of years it becomes increasingly difficult to maintain a healthy self-image. Limited mobility, limited income, and the undesirability of old age and waning health take their toll. The elderly grow to feel more and more isolated as friends die and events and activities fade deeper into the past.

Many older people have a great capacity for love at a time in life when, sadly, there are fewer people for them to care for and be cared by. They become sensitive to caring from people in their environment. Love is an action word. You express it nonverbally in what you do rather than in what you say.

The hurried, harried nurse who has time for nothing except nursing procedures, the one who cannot take the time to care about her patients as she tends to their care, would probably be happier in some other area of endeavor. It is certain that the elderly patients who would have to count on her for long-term care would be happier.

On a recent tour of The Palmcrest, a geriatric complex in Long Beach, California, a supervised residence, skilled nursing, and geriatric day-care facility, the director of nurses, Eleanor Johnson, R.N., illustrated a beautiful example of caring in action. On the way from one building to another, she was stopped by six patients; one to ask about his wife who was recuperating from a surgery in a nearby general hospital; another who wanted to tell Mrs. Johnson of her son's impending visit, and so it went. Each time she paused, spoke to the patient, always using his name, standing very close, looking directly at him, and touching him lightly on the hand or on the arm as she spoke. She seemed to have such an excellent instinct for nonverbal communication, because each time she stopped, she was saying to the patient nonverbally, "I am not too busy for you. You are important. I do care." In an interview that followed the tour, we asked if this was her usual practice. Mrs. Johnson replied:

> "Oh, yes. I always stop when one of the patients wants me to. I know that now is important to them. I never say later, unless there is an emergency and when there is, they also know that I'll be back as soon as I can. You know I hear nurses say it all the time, they just don't have time and can't stop every time a patient wants them to. But I don't agree. I think we can't afford not to stop. It takes me two minutes to walk over here and I imagine it took no more than four or five stopping as we did. What is a minute or two to me when it means so much to them."

It wasn't the amount of time she gave, it was the quality of that time.

The Palmcrest facility, under Mrs. Johnson's guidance, is outstanding. The buildings are bright, and cheerful, with no trace of nursing-home odor. All the patients who could be up were—on canes, walkers, or in wheelchairs; they were involved in activities of their choice out of the many offered. The facility has its own theater where movies and plays (put on by the local college drama department) are shown, the patients have their own band, choral group, art center and gallery, greenhouse, and shop where they sell their own art and crafts. The place is so stimulating that one enterprising eighty-four-year-old is taking a college course for credit. Outstanding as this facility is, its most impressive feature is the staff. They were all crisply neat, efficient, smiling, and pleasant. They relate to patients more like family members than caretakers. Eleanor Johnson attributes this to two factors:

> First of all, it isn't because we pay them any more money because we don't. I guess I just tell them how hard I have worked to achieve this environment for the patients and about

our reputation; that I want them to be just as proud as I am. We have a ninety-day probationary period and if I find a new employee, in any department, unkind, disrespectful, or neglectful of a patient, I fire him. But I think what is more important is I involve them in the patient care. We have staffings twice a week and we go over the patients' rehabilitation program. Maybe our goal is to get a patient to feed himself . . . or toilet trained . . . or out of his wheelchair, we all work toward that goal. We all get involved with the patient, we all care, and we all reap the tremendous inner rewards when the patient makes it.

Mrs. Johnson's explanation says a great deal and deserves more thought by all those who seek to improve the long-term care environment. But she forgot to mention one thing: modeling. When the professional nurse delivers excellent nursing care and treats her patients with humanity and dignity, she will have an excellent staff. She models, she sets the example. Conversely, if the professional nurse approaches her patients as things rather than as people, ridicules them, discusses their idiosyncrasies in front of others and is uncaring, her staff will follow suit. Geriatric patients' needs are not met by professional nurses alone, but they must assume the responsibility for teaching and for leading those others. Much of that leading and teaching will be done nonverbally, by setting a behavioral model for others to follow.

When dealing with older patients, nonverbal communication takes on added importance. We have already seen how love and caring are expressed in our behavior and how our nonverbal interactions will set an example for the semiskilled staff.

NURSING OBSERVATIONS IN GERIATRICS _____

We must also consider nursing observations that take on added importance in a geriatric setting because in many facilities there are no staff physicians, and private physicians visit irregularly. When the physician does visit, he will rely heavily on his patient's chart and the nursing notes which are a direct result of observations. Therefore, the geriatric nurse has an added responsibility that she would not have in an acute care facility where more medical personnel are involved in patient observation and evaluation. She also has an added advantage to help her with that responsibility. Since she is involved with the patient on a long-term basis, she knows him better and will be cued in more quickly by behavioral changes.

Mr. J., a 74-year-old CVA patient, had exhibited excellent rehabilitative progress during his 18-month hospitalization in an extended-care facility. He was able to feed and bathe himself and got around quite well with the help of a walker. He enjoyed the Saturday football game on TV, "visiting with the other folks," and almost nightly card games with a few select cronies. Suddenly, his energy waned. He was bedridden within a few weeks. The Director of Nurses was concerned and anxious for the physician's visit. When the doctor arrived, he checked Mr. J. carefully, ordered some routine tests that indicated no new complications and finally shook his head sadly, assuming that the degenerative process had sped up. However, one day, during a bed bath, an aide noticed that Mr. J.'s elbows were very hard. "The skin felt like a snake's," she reported to the director of nurses, who checked it out. The skin on the patient's elbows was very hard, which made the Director of Nurses suspect a possible thyroid deficiency. She called Mr. J.'s physician, explained the condition of the patient's elbows, and made some comments from the chart on his sudden change in behavior. The doctor ordered new tests, discovered thyroid deficiency, and prescribed a synthetic hormone. Mr. J. was soon able to resume his former mobility and activity. He remained at the facility until his death five years later. In Mr. J.'s case, nursing observations dramatically affected the quality of life during those last five years. The patient was able to live to the fullest of his capabilities. Observation resulted in a direct benefit to the patient.

Mr. J.'s nonverbal behavior was the cue, and the nurse's alert observation of that behavior resulted in the benefit. The physician had not been there on a daily basis as the nurse had to see Mr. J. going about the facility visiting, playing cards, and being involved.

The change in the patient's behavior was not observable to the physician, but it was to the nurse. She was open to the cue—in this case, the hard skin of the elbow, which she recognized as a symptom of thyroid deficiency. She did not shrug off the patient's behavior.

Simply stated, the nursing situation involves three things: the behavior of the patient, the nurse's reaction to that behavior, and the actions she takes for the patient's benefit. The final step, the action, is based on the first two interactions. Our understanding of nonverbal behavior allows us to be better nurses because we become better understanders. Our observations are more accurate. Often a nurse will have an inexplicable awareness that she will sometimes explain away as instinct or intuition. Actually, this awareness results from her direct observation of the patient's sudden change in behavior.

Since the patient and the nurse are both people, communication goes on between them, verbally and nonverbally. The patient also observes us and our behaviors. The older patient will probably be more trusting of his observations of our nonverbal behavior than he will of his understanding of our verbal communication. There are many reasons why. A large number of older people have lost hearing acuity, proficiency at speech, or have slowed down mentally. Even when they do not suffer from any of these impairments, there is still a gap of some fifty or sixty years that separates the young nurse from her aged patient. The same word might mean entirely different things to each of them.

Our vocabulary has changed in the past decade or two. A retired RN was recently glancing through a current issue of a nursing journal. She had trouble with some of the semantics and laughed, saying: "My goodness, things sure have changed since I was in nursing." How easy it would be to assume that because this patient was a nurse, she would automatically understand everything in a nursing journal. The assumption would not be correct, because nursing has changed, and she has not kept up with those changes. In many situations, the patient does not have the vocabulary to communicate with you. An 88-year-old retired train conductor might well have trouble finding a common vocabulary to converse with a 22-year-old BSN graduate.

Nonverbal communication can be used to increase understanding as a support to the spoken word. Paralanguage, as discussed in Chapter 1, deals with how something is said. When you have something pleasant to say to the patient, your smile (facial expression) helps him identify what is to be said as something pleasant. The following illustration could be used to demonstrate the point. The patient has undergone minor surgery for the removal of a tumor. On the nurse's first visit after surgery she commented that the tumor was benign and that everything was fine. The patient did not respond to her comment and seemed distraught. On checking the chart, the nurse learned that the patient, 79, was transferred from a long-term care facility for the surgery. The nurse can now make one of two assumptions: (1) The patient is confused, perhaps senile, and this accounts for his lack of response. (2) She can recognize the possibility that the patient did not understand her communication. If she makes the second assumption, she can go back to the patient's room, looking pleasant and cheerful and say to him: "When I was in earlier, you seemed upset. I thought I would come back and talk to you again. You know when I told you that the tumor was benign; that meant that the doctor did not find any trace of cancer. He cleaned the tumor out, so you should have no more trouble with that leg once the incision heals. Is there anything that you do not understand about the surgery or about what happens next, that I could help you with?"

This approach gives the patient the opportunity to comprehend his situation. Confusion can result when common medical terms and abbreviations are used. In this illustration, the patient did not understand the word "benign." The nurse's noncommittal facial expression added to the confusion, as the patient may have interpreted her expression as a sign of bad news, making it easier for him to assume that benign meant something else.

In a 1976 issue, *R.N. Magazine*[13] published an article on patients' understanding of common medical terms. The sampling included 200 adults, 50 percent of them high school graduates, 14 percent were college graduates, and an additional 21 percent with some college training. Only 51% of this sampling understood the word *benign.* These were not elderly, sometimes confused patients. The point is well taken. There is a need to use words appropriate to the patient's understanding and to accompany those words with nonverbal behaviors.

To establish a therapeutic environment, the nurse must develop a warm, friendly relationship with her geriatric patient, recognizing that her involvement with him is likely to be a long one. All too often, we are inclined to be judgmental of our elderly patients, writing them off as incontinent, senile, obstinate, or difficult. However, the patients judge us, too. They identify the grumpy nurse, the rough one, who is in too much of a hurry to care whether or not she hurts you, the phony who tells you one thing with her words and something quite different with her behavior. Patients judge you kindly when your behavior is effective, when you approach them cheerfully, when you allow them to show anger without making them feel guilty, when you allow them some decision in matters that concern them and when you give them options in their daily life. Patients judge you harshly when your behavior is ineffective, when you allow them to be alone for long periods of time, when you are abrupt and judgmental in your interactions, and when you say and do unkind things that reduce their self-esteem.

VALUES IN THE GERIATRIC SETTING

The humanistic values that most nurses possess should be used to improve geriatric medical care. A young RN who took a job at a geriatric facility was greeted her first day there by Mrs. T., the facility's difficult patient, who treated her to a ten-minute harangue on the personal and the professional ineptness of nurses in general and herself in particular. The abuse smarted; red-faced, the young nurse bit her tongue to avoid answering in kind. The other staff nurses had a good laugh and said: "That's our Mrs. T. She lets everybody have it. You'll get used to her." The young nurse couldn't get

Mrs. T. out of her mind, so she looked up her case and learned that Mrs. T. had been a successful attorney, was now widowed, with an only son who lived in a distant city. She was partially paralyzed with a neurogenic urinary disorder. Mrs. T. took no part in any of the facility's activities, preferring to stay alone in her private room. The nurse decided that she would make Mrs. T. her special project and asked the Director of Nurses if she could be assigned Mrs. T.'s nursing care during her shift. The DN agreed enthusiastically. The young nurse determined to break through to her patient, ignored the patient's volley of insults and rage. She did each procedure carefully, gently; answered the bell promptly and cheerfully. Within a few weeks, Mrs. T.'s attitude began to soften toward the nurse. She had fewer tantrums, and none when the young nurse was on duty. She was willing to talk sometimes and even began to smile occasionally, but Mrs. T. still refused to leave her room or to allow anyone to visit her there. One day, as the nurse was diapering Mrs. T., something came to her—an intuition, the awareness that comes from good observation. She realized that Mrs. T. was tense and close to tears and empathized with the problem that diapering must cause this independent lady. The nurse decided, with some trepidation, to get it out in the open.

"Mrs. T.," she began, "you seem very distressed about the diapers. If you are, maybe we can talk about it and find some way of handling the situation that will be more comfortable to you."

The patient put her head on the nurse's shoulder and wept. "You don't know how awful I feel," she finally said. "I'm so ashamed, just an old fool wetting my pants and having to wear diapers like a baby. I just don't want anyone to see me like this. I don't want anyone to know."

The young nurse took Mrs. T.'s problem to the DN, who agreed to try rubber pants with an insert. After some trial and error, Mrs. T. learned to handle her own changes without help; freed from what she saw as a shameful embarrassment, the patient's behavior improved. She made friends among the other patients and staff members; at last report, Mrs. T. is planning to write a book about her experiences as a young attorney during the 1920s and 1930s.

The nurse had not known Mrs. T. Her only experience was with the patient's behavior and the indirect information from others. However, she was not satisfied to write Mrs. T. off as simply hostile. She decided to break through to the patient. She did not take the insults personally, as, indeed, they were not meant personally. By her consistent posture of caring, the nurse won Mrs. T.'s trust. Here was a friend who could be trusted with the truth. Once the therapeutic environment was established, the nurse was able to benefit the patient. An alternate procedure to diapering was tried and, ultimately, allowed Mrs. T. to take care of herself, thereby restoring her self-esteem.

Having a problem should not be confused with being a problem. Some patients are diagnosed as hostile, confused, or senile and are written off to custodial care. Food, shelter, and sedation are provided, but little else. The geriatric nurse must learn to identify confusion, because the elderly are subject to many kinds of confusion, most of which can be dealt with. One patient may exhibit the symptoms of confusion resulting from hypoglycemia, whereas another patient's apparent confusion is caused by new and unfamiliar surroundings. Patients with hearing, visual, and speech impairments frequently appear confused, when in reality their difficulty is with verbal communication.

Deafness ranges from a mild loss of hearing to total deafness. People with impaired hearing react in different ways: some shout, others accuse people of mumbling or of trying to keep something from them; many become withdrawn and frequently appear confused. A patient charted as withdrawn and confused was unresponsive to everyone except one aide who always approached the patient directly, touching him lightly to get his attention and facing him directly as she spoke. In a staffing, she mentioned this to the Director of Nurses, explaining that this was the way she treated her own grandfather who was deaf. Tests were ordered for the patient, and he was found to have suffered a severe hearing loss. His apparent confusion was the result of his inability to hear what was being said to him.

If one loses his sight in youth or in middle age, other senses become overly developed to help compensate. Also, the person is still young enough to benefit from special training designed to teach him new ways of coping with his environment. But this is not true when a person loses his vision late in life. The other senses do not compensate and he may not be able to master mobility and other independent living skills. The elderly blind patient may appear confused; indeed, he often is confused in his efforts to relate to his environment. The patient who is both blind and hard of hearing has special difficulties communicating and interacting with others. Both blind and deaf patients can appear confused, but this confusion should not be mistaken for senility, because in most cases such patients can respond and benefit from rehabilitation.

Communication with patients who have had CVAs—cerebral hemorrhage, emboli, thromboses, or vascular insufficiencies—present special problems. The patient goes through an acute phase during which he is unconscious, and the prime concern is to keep him alive. But later, in the nursing facility, the patient begins the second phase, which is long-term rehabilitation. CVA patients often have difficulty communicating with both the spoken and the written word. The aphasic patient loses all ability with words. This decreased ability to communicate is frequently but incorrectly viewed as a symptom of mental illness, or a lack of intelligence. One of the causes of this difficulty is hardening of the arteries (arteriosclerosis), which affects the circulation of blood to the speech center of the brain. In many cases, the patient knows what he wants to say but is unable to say it, or thinks that he has said it and does not know why the nurse is not responding. Sometimes, stroke victims entirely lose certain words and can no longer grasp things they once understood. Gaps develop in the conversation, as the patient only partially understands. Some people will try to cover this gap by smiling, nodding in agreement, or becoming aggressive. When the patient does not understand what is being said, he will fill in the empty spaces. He will do this by coming in on nonverbal communicative levels. Therefore, a great deal of business between nurse and the patient must be done nonverbally. When you speak to the patient or give him instructions, be sure that he is looking at you and let your face reflect what you are saying. Touch him to get his attention, offer him your arm when you wish to lead him somewhere, use gestures whenever you think they are needed, and do not be afraid to repeat your gestures and words until they are understood. We use pictures to help young children understand, and pictures will sometimes be helpful with CVA patients.

A CVA patient once said, "I remember talking to my son, then suddenly time stood still in the middle of a thought." The patient was sane; he could still think. His difficulty was in communicating those thoughts. It is tremendously important to the rehabilitation of stroke patients that they be assured that they are not thought of as dumb or demented.

Since older people have a need to feel useful and valued, they can fill that need by helping each other. One facility places newly arrived CVA patients as roommates to other CVA patients who have progressed well in their rehabilitation. The DN always talks to the person first, explaining that the new patient has had the same illness. She is careful how she matches the patients, and in most cases it has been successful, with the healthier patient helping the sicker one along the rough road to rehabilitation.

There are other ways to provide peer support in a long-term care facility. Those with good vision can read to the blind and near-blind, take them for walks. They can teach each other skills. Someone who is trying to master a walker may learn more quickly with a few tips from another patient who has recently learned himself. An 88-year-old lady never misses a meal in the dining room because her friend needs her there to cut her meat.

GERIATRICS IN THE ACUTE CARE FACILITY _____

The full-time geriatric nurse is a specialist and needs special qualities. She must be capable of mature judgment, empathic and loving; she must be soundly instructed in the disease of old age and skilled in the requisite nursing procedures. In no other area of nursing will her role be so versatile. She will be a social worker, dietician, teacher, recreation director, counselor, speech therapist, physiotherapist, and, above all, friend. She will use all her abilities in her many roles and frequently will call on her own private well of imagination and humor.

The geriatric specialist has a wide choice of working areas because geriatric nursing is done in acute-care hospitals, skilled nursing facilities, long-term nursing homes, in private duty, and through restorative home health care. Acute-care hospitals are not ideally suited for long-term care, especially for geriatric patients. They do not have available space to provide a setting for the activities and socialization; they are geared to treat acute rather than chronic health problems, and they do not have adequate staff to help the older patient relearn or maintain his living skills. Therefore, acute-care hospitals are likely to foster dependency by treating the geriatric patient in the same manner as the short-term acute-care patient. Rehabilitation is frequently measured in the same terms as it is for younger patients. For example, an elderly stroke victim's newly learned ability to feed himself may not be viewed as a positive rehabilitative step. The economic factor also contributes to the problem of long-term geriatric care; even with governmental and private health insurance, acute hospitalization is too expensive for most elderly patients. Elderly patients in acute-care facilities require special consid-erations. An 80-year-old, for example, falls and breaks his hip. He is brought by ambulance to the emergency room of a general hospital, where the nurse tries to get admission information from him. The patient may appear confused or respond inappro-priately. His confusion can be the result of pain and fear, or simply because of a hearing loss which makes it difficult for him to understand the nurse's questions. He will probably not respond the same as an 18-year-old or a 40-year-old would with a similar fracture and, indeed, his physical condition may be much worse because of a preexisting condition, such as diabetes or cardiac complications. If the nurse is understanding and a keen observer, she will be able to help the patient to cope.

Staff nurses will face many of the same situations. A stroke patient may be hospital-ized for cataract surgery. A viable nursing care plan will have to include care for the preexisting stroke, as well as the recent surgery. We become very used to doing things for acute-care patients and with an older, apparently frail person, we are inclined to do everything for him instead of helping the patient to help himself. It is better to let the patient do everything he can for himself, as long as it is not potentially dangerous to himself or to others.

Even nursing students who do not intend to specialize in geriatrics should take some additional time to study and to understand the multiple problems of old age. Roughly 20 percent of general hospital admissions are over 65, and that figure is bound to rise with the growing geriatric population. Their stay in a general hospital may be for a short-term, but that does not mean that the quality of their nursing care should be diminished. Therefore, students should have courses in geriatric nursing, which deal with the physical needs of the elderly patient, and in gerontology—which deals with aging, emphasizing the socioeconomic and psychological factors.

Geriatric Home Health Care

A great majority of people with chronic illness are in the older age groups and older people, given the right circumstances, seem to do better in their own homes among family and familiar surroundings. As a person becomes older, it is more difficult to adjust to new surroundings, and change can be traumatic. Therefore, home health nursing provides a means for keeping older people with chronic health problems at home. But those nurses working in home health care, or restorative home health care, will have to deal with some situations that are beyond the bounds of what is normally recognized as skilled nursing care. The home health nurse will have to assess the patient's role in the home, the presence or absence of other people, and the supportive or detrimental attitude of those others. She will have to consider safety and security factors. And she will have to determine that the patient's illness can be treated and his level of health maintained in the home environment.

Home health nurses identify the need for support systems to help people maintain themselves at home. An elderly woman living by herself may need the services of a homemaker several times a week. For a patient with poor vision, the nurse may need to print in large letters a sheet of medication instructions to be tacked to the door of the medicine cabinet. Some patients will need protective wearing apparel, while others will need special tableware so that they can feed themselves without fear of breaking, spilling, or dropping. Unlike the hospital setting, making arrangements for these items will entail more than a call to central service on the nurse's part.

Even in the home, the elderly chronically ill patient suffers from stresses that can be lessened when the visiting nurse uses her skills to help the patient to maintain a sense of constancy. The patient should be allowed as much control over his environment as possible and should not be restricted in his activity unless it is absolutely necessary. Sometimes we fear that our older patients will injure themselves, and this fear leads us to be too restrictive. We deprive the individual of his freedom when we really do not have to. A walk to the corner with a cane, for example, does present some risk. The patient may fall and complicate his condition with a fractured or broken bone, but the hazard must be weighed against the probable depression that may be caused by depriving the patient of a previously enjoyed pleasure. In some situations you will approve, even encourage the daily walk, while in others you will decide that the patient is just too shaky on his feet and veto the walk. Whenever you do have to restrict the patient from enjoying some activity, try to find something else that he can do safely. Time hangs heavy for the elderly, and an additional void will exist if the patient is deprived of an activity and left with nothing to take its place. Finding an active listener will be an invaluable aid. If you have really listened to your patient, you will know something about his personality and maybe even have had a few hints as to what he likes to do.

Because of illness or diminished capacities, your patient may lose his previous opportunity for socialization. While you should encourage him to socialize, you must be astute enough to recognize the problems caused by poor hearing, speech, vision, mobility, or bladder control and help the patient find ways to circumvent these problems so that he does not become homebound.

The home health nurse has the same primary problem that all nurses have—time. Because of scheduling, there is a limit to the quantity of time that can be spent with each patient. However, the quality of that time can be enhanced by the intelligent application of nonverbal techniques. The nurse who visits in the home becomes important to the patient. If she appears disinterested or uncaring, she contributes to the patient's depression and alienation from the rest of society. Here is yet another person to whom he has become a bother. The patient will not trust the nurse or give her his confidence. He may express these feelings by withdrawing and by giving her the silent treatment, or try to outfox her by lying about taking his medication, feigning the severity of his pain. When a patient behaves this way, the nurse becomes totally ineffective, regardless of the excellence of her nursing techniques. She has failed to interact therapeutically with the patient and will not be able to benefit him until trust and confidence are restored.

But the nurse who approaches the patient in a friendly manner, chats with him, listens to what he says, is gentle in her treatment of his person and considerate of his surroundings and belongings, wins the patient's confidence. For some, her visit will become the highlight of the week. A therapeutic environment will be created because of mutual trust, and the patient will confide that he forgot his medication, fell again, or had severe pain. Then the visiting nurse will be effective because she will be able to meet the patient's true needs.

SKILLED NURSING FACILITIES _____

We sometimes wonder why poor-quality nursing homes are not closed. Perhaps the main reason that they are not is that we do not have enough space to meet the needs of the elderly, and those elderly people who rely on them would have no place to go if they were closed. It may not be possible or even advisable to institutionalize all of our elderly who are partially incapacitated by chronic medical problems. Alternatives certainly are available to us, and home health care may be a viable one for many. It allows the older person to remain in his social and home environment. Home health costs are fractional in comparison to acute and extended care. In the near future, we may see tremendous growth in this field of nursing, which presents a humane alternative to permanent hospitalization for the elderly.

Home health care and acute-care hospital nurses do care for a certain number of geriatric patients, but the primary environment for geriatric nursing is in a skilled nursing facility. For the purposes of this text, when we speak of skilled nursing facility (SNF), we mean any long-term nursing provider, including nursing homes and convalescent hospitals. Many nurses who do not dislike geriatrics do dislike some of these facilities.

Many older people tend to deteriorate rapidly once they enter a nursing home. A walk through a poorly run nursing home gives evidence of the reason why, as we see elderly patients in bed or sitting around, poorly groomed, in an aroma of feces and urine, with little evidence of professional nursing care; patients are dull-eyed from loss of hope or, in some cases, from sedation that has been used too freely. Is this why we do not like geriatric settings? Is this the only road open?

Skilled nursing facilities should not be just custodial centers for the aged. Ideally, they should meet the needs for long-term patient care, but they must also be concerned with life setting, basic living skills, social interaction, and the psychological needs of the patients. They must create a home that will be, for many patients, their last home.

Some SNF patients will be younger, recuperating from surgeries, fractures, or strokes —patients who no longer require acute medical–surgical care, but who are not yet ready to return home. These patients will stay several weeks or months, then they will be discharged. But the largest population in SNFs will continue to be our older citizens, many of whom will never return home and who will spend the rest of their lives in the institution.

These are the patients who present the greatest challenge. They are very much with us, even though we sometimes do not like to think about them, and they need compassionate, professional nursing.

People are admitted to SNFs for various reasons, but they all share a common need for care. Perhaps one person only needs help because he cannot manage on his own and there is no one to help him, while another needs total nursing care and is unable to function outside the SNF. The nurse will encounter all kinds of patients with vastly different pathologies. Within the same hour, you may care for an aphasic patient who needs constant care and the spry 85-year-old who is still alert but who is unable to manage on his own. These patients will have different medical needs, and different personal, social, and psychological needs. The geriatric nurse will be involved with the needs of both.

In the SNF setting, the nurse not only deals with the disease but with its effects, which can be so overwhelming that the patient can no longer be maintained in a normal home environment.

When we speak of improving the quality in SNFs, we too often mean quality in terms of acute care—more and better procedures, more medication, more paperwork—rather than in terms of improving the quality of life. Improved quality should be viewed in terms of better use of the facility and of making that facility more livable to the people whose home it has become. Proxemics, which is generally considered to be man's perception of his social and personal space, is involved in the livability of the facility. Studies in recent years have pointed to the therapeutic value of proxemics (environment) on behavior and self-concept of the long-term patient. Facilities are inspected for safety and cleanliness, but seldom is any thought given to the livability of the facility.

For instance, beds are set at prescribed angles in prescribed locations, with no consideration of the patients' preference. A nurse who understands proxemics will be sympathetic to the patient's need to have personal things around him and will tolerate the occasional clutter. She can serve as a model for the nonprofessional health care deliverers by showing sensitivity toward the possessions and privacy of others by saying such things as, "May I come in," when entering a patient's room and, "Do you mind if I move this?" when rearranging his things. She will discuss daily living plans with the patient and will allow him to make decisions whenever possible. She will recognize the importance of the SNF's atmosphere and will know that it consists of the attitudes of people, as well as the physical surroundings.

Those attitudes can be caring and constructive, or indifferent and destructive. In his own home, the patient creates his atmosphere. He surrounds himself with the things he knows and loves, and invites into his personal territory the people he knows and loves. But in the long-term facility, his territory is created by someone else. A good atmosphere does not just happen. It is the result of a great deal of the right kind of effort on the part of someone with the empathy and skill to create it.

Effective Geriatric Care

We are all familiar with the "whole person" concept, and nowhere in nursing is it more important than in the SNF, where a nurse must respond to all the patient's needs. The challenges are varied and presented daily if not hourly.

Frequently, the nurse will find herself acting as the patient's advocate and presenting the patient's cause to administration. Mobility might be in question, as many SNFs discourage mobility for fear that the patient will wander off or fall and hurt himself; because of this, many patients lead lives far more restricted than their physical limitations would necessitate. They are often kept in one place by means of medication and restraints, and that one place is bed. Yet, for the elderly patient to live life fully, he should be able to enjoy the maximum degree of mobility. Patient restrictions are not always an indication of callousness on the part of administration. Many restrictions are merely the result of what appears to be the best way to cope with a possible danger. The effective geriatric nurse will work with the admisistration toward developing more humane solutions that are in keeping with good medical procedures and in full consideration of the needs of the whole patient.

The quality of care also needs to be improved in the area of diagnosis. Nurses are often told that a patient's condition is simply due to old age when, in fact, a better diagnosis could be made. Nurses need an accurate diagnosis to formulate valid care plans. Thoughtful diagnosis must be included as a component in upgrading the quality of SNF care. Nurses make their contribution to this improvement by careful and accurate patient observation.

Effective geriatric nursing means that the nurse has the skills to provide good nursing care, the empathy to understand the patient, the desire to help him, and the nonverbal techniques to interact with him therapeutically. The geriatric nurse must be concerned with extending the patient's life, and she must be equally concerned with the quality of life.

6
Death and Dying

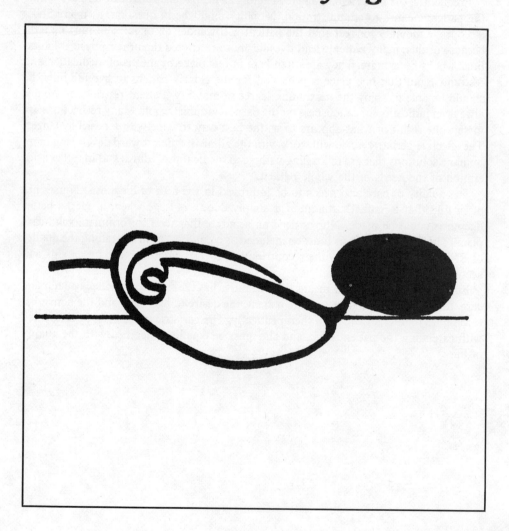

THE WORLD OF THE DYING PATIENT _____

Evelyn lay dying. There was no doubt that she was dying. She knew this final reality that had become her only reality. An orderly stuck his head past the partially opened door. "Is the charge nurse here?" He saw that she was not, and disappeared without waiting for or expecting an answer. Evelyn looked over to the empty bed of her former roommate, Mae, who had died many weeks ago—or was it only a day or two past? Evelyn really didn't know or care. Time—at least that kind of time—didn't matter any more. She only knew that she had lost the last friend of her eighty-two years. Now, she was alone.

Where was it? . . . yes, that was it—she had read many years before when she was a girl about the Eskimos who, when they were too old or too sick or too laden with human sorrow, when . . . how did they express it? . . . "When life is heavier than death," they did not hesitate to end it and cross into the distant land. And how they did it. She remembered that in some tribes they would throw a great party; everyone would have a grand time, and in the midst of the gaiety, the oldster would ask his favorite son or daughter to put the rope around his neck and to hoist him to his death. Not a bad way to go, Evelyn thought, surrounded by people and by love and by laughter. Of course, for her, there was no favorite son or daughter, for she bore the great sorrow of having outlived all her children.

The nurse came in to change Evelyn's soiled bed. "I told you to ring for the bedpan. Why can't you do what I tell you? . . . this is the third time today." Evelyn stared wordlessly at the ceiling and set herself to receive the shock of pain that accompanied any movement. She hated this nurse who was too great a fool to know that she would have rung the bell if she could ever tell it was going to happen before it happened.

Evelyn slept for awhile. When she woke, the charge nurse was there. She didn't know her name, but she was awfully nice and always stopped for a moment at her bedside. Sometimes, she would sit for a few minutes while she wrote on the chartboard. She would always say something to Evelyn, hold her hand or stroke her forehead . . . occasionally, she could stay and read to her for a few minutes . . . or tell her about the newly arrived spring . . . the sun on the mountains which Evelyn could no longer see for herself. She never spoke to the charge nurse, but by gesture of her hand or a movement of her eyes she let her know what she wanted, and the charge nurse always knew just as if she could read Evelyn's mind. She knew because she cared.

Evelyn never spoke to this nurse whom she had come to love and thought to herself some day I must say "thank you" to her. Then she remembered that she could not speak and so she smiled . . . a distorted grimace with a good side of her face that had to say all the "thank you's" of her heart. Life was heavier than death, but death is so difficult.

The world of the dying patient is one that we enter reluctantly, if at all. And this is understandable. Doctors, nurses—all health care specialists—are devoted to saving life and to the restoration of health. To many of us, the dying patient is almost an affront to our profession. We speak of "losing the patient," or of Dr. So and So's "coronary" not making it. The disease has won and, despite our best efforts, we have lost. Death has defeated us professionally, just as it will ultimately claim us personally. When we look at the pale lifeless face of a patient who has just died, we cannot help but recognize the full measure of our mortality. Yet death is the final step, and, for an ever-increasing number of people, it will occur in an acute or a skilled nursing facility. As a nurse, you will be involved with dying patients, and no amount of personal aversion will alter this fact.

What do we really know about death? Until recently, very little that would help us professionally. True, theologians have dealt with it, and it has been the theme from many pulpits, but generally in terms of salvation and immortality. Writers and poets have spoken of death. "I could lay down like a tired child, And weep away the life of care, Which I have borne and must yet bear, Till death like sleep might steal on me." Beautiful as it is, Shelley's quote says little that will help a nurse cope with a dying patient and his grieving family.

During the past decade, important work has been done in the area of the "death crisis." Research and clinical studies have given us a new insight into the special world of the dying patient.

These insights can be of invaluable help to the professional nurse. A new methodology will doubtlessly emerge from these studies and insights. Thanatology, from Thanatos meaning death is the study of death & dying, may eventually become a discipline in nursing curricula. But let us hope that it will never be reduced to an automatized technique, because this would be no great improvement over what patients have had to contend with during recent years. All interactions with terminally ill patients must be honed by our own humanity because, just as surely as no two people live the same kind of lives, no two people die the same kind of deaths.

Humanity is the key word, and most nurses are superbly equipped to deal with the terminally ill. They have all the right instincts, and only need a little understanding and a strong memory of what caused them to decide on a nursing career in the first place. Usually, it was a desire to help others. Unfortunately, that original desire is frequently disciplined into the background in the urgency forced on students to master the technical aspects of nursing.

Since this text is on nonverbal communication, most of the material covered in this chapter will be concerned with the identification and value of nonverbal exchanges and cues in the world of the dying patient. However, to promote a broader understanding, we will first review some of the more important studies that have influenced our changing attitudes and approach to the dying patient.

SOME RECENT STUDIES ON DEATH AND DYING _____

During the late 1960s, psychologist Morton A. Lieberman[14] was conducting a study of geriatric patients in an extended care facility. He noted that one of the nurses working there had an uncanny ability. She seemed remarkably accurate in predicting the impending death of elderly patients several months in advance and before there were any physical indications that death was imminent. The nurse was unable to explain what led to her predictions, except that a patient approaching death just seemed to act differently.

Lieberman was intrigued with the phenomenon, and decided to administer psychotests to a selected group of elderly patients to see if identifiable psychological changes did, indeed, occur as death approached. In this study, Lieberman required each of the subjects to perform a series of tasks, and he later found that several of these were related to the imminence of death. Two of these tests, which he has specifically cited, were the Bender–Gestalt test. In this, the patient is asked to draw, freehand, copies of geometric figures. In the second study, the same subjects were asked to draw a person. Both of these tests were administered to a group of 30 elderly volunteers every three to four weeks over a period of two years. None of these volunteers was suffering from an incapacitating physical or mental disorder. Five of the subjects dropped out or died before the study was completed.

The variables in this study that related to the imminence of death were (1) ego energy, based on the size of the freehand drawings of the Bender–Gestalt figures; (2) ego sufficiency, based on the complexity of the human figure drawings; (3) organization–disorganization, based on the adequacy of the Bender–Gestalt figures. These tests were administered to all the subjects at least five times, and subjects who died less than three months after completing the fifth and the final study were placed in the death imminent (DI) group. Subjects who were still alive one year after the tests were placed in the death delayed (DD) group. (Lieberman, "Psychological Evaluations of Impending Death: Some Preliminary Evaluations," *Journal of Gerontology* 20(2), pp. 189–90.)

An immediate and logical guess would be that the D.I. group would be lower on all the measures than the D.D. group. It is reasonable to assume that those who died shortly after completing the tests would be lower on ego energy, sufficiency, and organization than those who remained alive longer. However, this was not found to be the case, and Lieberman's study indicated that nearness to death did not bring about psychological change. The problems that the aged go through in facing death may have more to do with coping than the imminence of death itself. Fear of death and psychological change during the last months of life may result from a crisis in the environment and may not be due to lack of resolution of the death question. Lieberman found that many of his elderly subjects had worked out the meaning of death for themselves and were quite willing to talk about it. The individual's background had a great deal to do with his acceptance or lack of it. People living at home with families and those in other supportive environments usually did better. As death approaches, environment may be the key factor in the psychological changes that occur in so many people.

Lieberman's work was conducted in an extended care setting with aged patients and may, therefore, provide insight only as far as the geriatric nursing experience is concerned. Children, the young, and middle-aged die as well and, in an acute-care facility, we are likely to meet death in all age groups. Dr. Elisabeth Kübler-Ross conducted a hospital-centered study with dying patients; the findings of her study has powerfully affected current concepts of nursing.

Dr. Kübler-Ross on Death and Dying

Dr. Kübler-Ross was approached by a group of young theology students who had been assigned to write a paper on crisis. They determined that death was man's greatest crisis and solicited the aid of Dr. Kübler-Ross in researching material for the paper. There was no precedent for research on this subject, so the students and Dr. Kübler-Ross decided that: The best way to study death and dying would be to ask the patients themselves (Kübler-Ross, *On Death and Dying*).[15] They would observe the critically ill patients, study their responses and needs, evaluate their reactions to people around them, and get just as close to the dying as they would allow.

Reaching the first patient proved difficult, as doctors and nurses turned away from Dr. Kübler-Ross in stunned disbelief and anger. "Do you enjoy telling a 20-year-old man that he has only a couple of weeks to live?" was the irate response of one young nurse who walked hastily away before Dr. Kübler-Ross could explain the project. This young nurse may have said a great deal more than she meant to say. Her young patient's imminent death was unacceptable to her; perhaps she was unable to come to grips with her own feelings, or could not face the fact that all of her skills were ineffectual and she could do nothing to save the life of her patient, whose life should have been just beginning and not ending. In either case, it is doubtful that she could reach beyond her own feelings to give her patient the support he needed to face his final crisis.

Dr. Kübler-Ross interviewed over 200 terminally ill patients and identified five stages of dying. When nursing critically ill patients, you may encounter these stages sequentially very much as they are described here, or isolated in one of the stages.

Denial

Most patients, when told that they have a terminal illness, react by first denying the prognosis. They think, "No, not me. It can't be true." Some will insist that their report was mixed up with another patient's and will demand new tests; others will go doctor hunting in the usually vain hope of finding a more optimistic diagnosis. There is a need to face death and to cope with the reality of it. But in the early stages, denial is helpful to the patient; it is a buffer that protects him from the shock and allows him necessary time to reorganize his psyche. The patient should never be forced into a discussion of his impending end, and especially not when the news is fresh. If your patient should say to you, "No, it can't be me, I won't believe it," you will not help him by insisting that it is, indeed, him, that his disease is terminal, and he might as well face it. The patient must not be forced into someones else's timetable. He will begin to talk about it when he is ready, and not when you feel he should be ready.

When the patient insists that he is not the one, silence can be helpful, since it neither reinforces the denial nor impinges on the patient's need for denial. Silence used in this circumstance should be accompanied by other nonverbal behaviors, such as eye contact with the patient or a gesture such as hand holding. Use your silence effectively. Do not interpret using silence to mean that you should ignore the question and walk away from the patient. Let your silence say, "I am here, I will help you any way I can, you are not alone."

With few exceptions, denial is a temporary defense and will be replaced by partial acceptance and, finally, acceptance.

Anger

Dr. Kübler-Ross sees the second stage of dying as anger. Denial that can no longer be maintained is generally replaced by anger. "Why me?" the patient thinks to himself, and looks at someone else thinking, "Why not him instead of me?" To some, death is life's final low blow. The patient never achieved the business position he wanted . . . was never able to buy a new car or take that long-planned vacation . . . went bald young, and here he is now dying before his time . . . or before he is ready . . . or in too much pain. He is angry. The angry patient is difficult and frequently vocal. The nurses are bad, the doctors fools, and the food rotten. The poor nurse gives this patient her best effort and is repaid with sarcasm, curses, shouting, or silent hostility. We take this anger personally too often, and respond accordingly. His bell is answered last, and we do not go in at all if it is not ringing. It is hard to cope with angry patients. But where does that anger come from? Is the patient really angry at us? Wouldn't we be angry, too? The patient sees the staff bustling around in apparent good health, off to home and family after the day's work, while he realizes he may never go home again. We cannot take his anger personally when we understand it, because that angry patient is the someone who needs us . . . the someone to help—the one who first motivated us into a nursing career. Once you understand his anger, you will be able to give the patient respect and time. His tantrums will stop; his voice will be lowered, and the curses will cease. While this patient is exhibiting anger, he is frightened. When that anger subsides, he will need someone there who will listen and care. During his angry phase, your nonverbal language will speak to him louder than your words. It will state or deny that you are a caring someone who will be there. Think of some of the areas mentioned in Chapter 1 as you interact with critically ill patients. What is your facial expression? Do you approach this patient with tight-lipped determination? Do you keep your body stiff and tense in his presence, chart his vital signs as quickly as possible, so that you can get out of the room before he has a chance to make another comment on your poor nursing care? If you do, you are taking the patient's anger personally and responding to it, which can only make his already desperate situation more difficult.

Bargaining

Bargaining is the third stage explained by Dr. Kübler-Ross. In its basic form, bargaining is something we all use. "I'll do this for you, if you will do such and such for me." The child pleads with the parent that he will be very good and do everything asked, if he can only have the desired new toy. Many dying patients bargain. One may promise to accept death graciously, if he can just live to see a grandchild born . . . a son graduated from college . . . his wife reconciled. Bargaining is not always for an extension of life; sometimes it is for a period free of pain or the ability to meet death lucidly and with dignity. But most often, it is for extended life. The critically ill person may promise to turn over a new leaf and dedicate his life to good works if he is spared. But death is not a punishment. It is the ultimate end for us all; it will not be bought off with good works.

Some patients have unfinished business; they grieve over some of the errors of their lives and bargain for enough time to right them. For example, a middle-aged woman married to a loving man, the mother of three grown children, suddenly spoke to her husband of her first child born before their marriage and given up for adoption. The husband had never known, but managed to control his own feelings and began contacting the agencies involved in an attempt to locate his wife's child before it was too late. Our personal value system might label this patient's behavior selfish and destructive. Why add to the grief of her family by dredging up the memory of the long-forgotten child? Why add to the tragedy and hurt her family were already facing? The patient had a very real need to make peace with her relinquished child. Bargaining is not as easy to identify as denial and anger, but it is equally as real. Active listening and empathy are two of our most effective nonverbal behaviors during the bargaining stage. Through active listening, we will know the patient's unfinished business and may be able to help him work it through. Since death is the final confrontation with our own mortality, nothing is too inconsequential if it helps us to put things in order and see the value of our lives.

Grieving

Kübler-Ross's fourth stage is depression or grieving. The patient can no longer deny his illness, and he suffers the grief of having to prepare for his final separation from the world. He is losing all that he loves, including his own life. This is not self-pity, but true grief; the patient in this stage should not be told to be stoic and to think only of his family. He has the right to think of himself, and he has the right to grieve for himself. As we have discussed earlier, your nonverbal communications are invaluable in caring for someone during the dying stages. This is especially true of the fourth stage. Words appeal to the intellect, and nonverbal behavior is more clearly understood emotionally. During the grieving stage, the person is preparing for the final separation and is reacting with his emotions. Nonverbal communications will give him the most comfort. He needs an active listener who is willing to just listen, to be near, and to accept his depression and his grief, someone to touch him gently.

Acceptance

The final stage is acceptance. Given enough time and some help in working through the other stages, the patient will reach a point where he is neither angry nor depressed. He will have mourned the impending loss of so many loved people and places. "He will contemplate his coming end with a certain degree of quiet expectation." (Kübler-Ross, *On Death and Dying*) This stage should not be seen as a period of happiness, since it is a period almost devoid of feeling. The struggle is over, and the time has come for the final rest.

THE SPECIAL NEEDS OF TERMINAL PATIENTS _____

Terminally ill patients do have special needs that we can understand and that we can meet if we take the time to understand. A great many of these needs will be satisfied nonverbally through empathetic nursing care. Kübler-Ross has stressed the importance of nonverbal cues and interactions in dealing with critically ill patients, and she feels that the psychological impact of nonverbal communications on the dying patient cannot be underrated.

Your closeness to the patient and your willingness to talk to him even though he may not be able to reply tells him that you care and that he is still a full human being worthy of your time and attention.

Many terminal patients are unable to reply or to respond. Communication with the dying, aphasic patient can be difficult. These patients are only able to communicate with you nonverbally; you will learn to interpret their symbols with a little time and practice. Sometimes, the patient is able to write with a pencil in his mouth. With other aphasic patients you can work out a symbol for "yes" and one for "no"; the patient can, for example, squeeze your hand—one squeeze means "yes" and two means "no." Eye blinks will work just as well. Once your symbolic system of blinks or hand squeezes is worked out and understood by the patient, anticipate questions so that the patient may respond with the newly worked-out system. The patient will be responding to you exclusively with nonverbal cues, while you will be able to combine speech and nonverbal cues. Your monologue with the patient might go something like this: "Are you comfortable?" The patient responds with two blinks for "no." "Are you in pain?" And again the two blinks. "Are you cold?" This time, the patient blinks once for "yes." Now you know, and the relatively little time this procedure has taken is nothing to compare to the joy of being able to know the aphasic patient's need and to satisfy it. How simple! A pair of bed socks or an extra blanket and he will be comfortable and more secure because he has found a means of communicating with you.

The monologue is not always so simple. You can run out of direct questions and not be able to find the one that the patient so desperately wants to answer. All you can do is to explain that you are trying and will stay with it. You could then suggest to the patient that you are going to try categories and that he should give you a "yes" response when you come to the right one. Your monologue would then proceed along the lines of: "Is it about your family, someone here at the hospital, do you want something from home, do you want me to telephone someone for you?" and so on until you come to the right subject. It may not be possible to find the right question in one session. Ask the patient if it is urgent, and when it is either stay or find someone else to continue working with him until the question has been identified and answered. After the symbols for communication have been worked out with the patient, all staff members dealing with him should be made aware of his newly established means of communication. The charge nurse should be informed so she can make the appropriate entry on the patient's nursing care plan.

There are times when you cannot respond to the patient's symbolic language quickly enough, but all you can do is try. You might make a mistake in interpretation; the patient will still know that you are doing your best, and he may find a clearer way to express his need.

Frequently, you come into contact with a patient, especially in CCU and ICU, who was stricken at home. His first realization comes in the hospital where he finds himself hooked up to various life-saving devices that make it impossible for him to speak. Paper and pencil will probably not be readily available, so you must become aware of the patient's eye movement and expressions. Spend a little extra time with him to find out what cues he is giving you and try to respond to them. He may not be able to speak, but he can hear. Tell him where he is, who you are, what the equipment is for, when his doctor was there, and when he is coming back. If your own shift has just started, tell him that you will be there for the next eight hours; you will come by his bed often; you will never be far away; and he is not alone. Sit by his bed for a few moments to reinforce what you have just said. This procedure is also helpful in dealing with intubated patients who are usually afraid of asphyxiation. Here again, you must look at the eyes. When they express fear go ahead and say: "Are you afraid?" Patient will generally indicate that he is, so stay by him for a few minutes asking, are you afraid of a, b, c, d? When he responds to one of the examples, explain what is happening, calm him and stay by him, or get someone else to until he has overcome the worst of his fear and anxiety.

It is rather generally believed that the last sense to fail before death is hearing and, if this is true, we can continue to communicate to the dying patient, even when he is no longer able to respond. What we say and how we touch him will be the last things he carries out of this world with him. A once vigorous man lay dying, comatose, of cancer. His illness had developed rapidly since the previous year when he and his family first learned of it. The elderly parents were called from a distant city to be there for the last and arrived in time to live their son's dying day. One of the staff nurses was about to bathe the patient when the family arrived. Instead, she said to him softly, "Dan, your parents are here." She explained that she was about to bathe and shave their son and asked if they would like to help. They said they would, and she guided them through the procedure. The nurse left for a few minutes and returned with coffee and told the family that they would not have to observe visiting hours, could stay for as long as they wished, and that she would be there to help whenever they needed her. She checked the respirator, moistened the patient's mouth, spoke to him gently of what she was doing and of the presence of his family. Then she got chairs for the elderly couple and told them that even though the patient could not speak or respond to them, there was a very good chance that he could hear, so they should speak to him of the things they wished to say. Throughout her shift, this caring nurse was never far away and when it ended, she stayed on, checking paper work, any excuse to stay because she felt the end was very near, the parents were used to her and would be comforted by her presence. The patient expired an hour later.

Most nurses are superbly equipped to deal with the terminally ill. They have all the right instincts. All they need is a little understanding and a strong remembrance of what was in their hearts that caused them to decide on a career in nursing.

This nurse spoke eloquently of care, caring not only for the dying patient but for his grieving family. She never said, "I really care," but she did say it many times nonverbally by her gentle touching of the patient, her concern in keeping his mouth and nose moist, her willingness to be the someone close by when the family faced the final moment.

Where Do We Begin?

How does one learn? You start by understanding yourself and your own feelings about death and dying people. You think about the kind of care you would want for yourself and your loved ones and through this develop empathy for those who are going through the death crisis.

You learn by being honest with yourself and trying to learn what kind of a nurse you really want to be, and, most important, you will learn from your patients if you take the time to understand their verbal and nonverbal behaviors.

A nurse, who we will call Nurse Mary, worked as a surgical nurse for over fifteen years in a large metropolitan hospital, then decided to take semiretirement in a small community where her husband had purchased a small farm. To supplement the family income, Nurse Mary went back to work. The only available job was as charge nurse in an extended care facility. She took the job and ran the hospital like a well-drilled marine troop, and the patients played the role she assigned them, namely, that of the good patient. Anger and hostility were punished with tight-lipped lectures, and the dying were told to cheer up, that they would probably live forever. Under her guidance, the facility was spotlessly clean, and the nursing care above reproach, but most of her elderly patients were depressed, and some had even drawn into silent isolation. Mary was a good nurse. She had met death many times in her surgical career, but never on a personal basis. The anesthesized patient was a surgical procedure to her, and she knew nothing of the patient as a person with hopes and dreams and fears. She was insulated by her total involvement with the procedure, so when she was forced to meet death on a personal basis with patients, many of whom she had come to love, she was unable to face it. Her case is not ususual. Nothing in her training, or the career that followed, had prepared her to handle these situations. Like many nursing students, she had been thrust into the hospital with no preparation for treating the dying patient.

Like Nurse Mary, Joy Ufema, R.N., of the Harrisburg Hospital, Harrisburg, Pennsylvania, was ill prepared to cope with the hospitalized, terminal patient. But Ms. Ufema began to notice the abysmal treatment of these patients. After a great deal of soul-searching, she went to her supervisor and asked to be assigned to the hospital's dying patients. The supervisor, to Ms. Ufema's surprise, agreed and, for the past five years, Joy Ufema has worked with these patients. She has written articles for *The Journal of American Nursing* and is involved in other projects that are designed to improve the environment of the dying. We asked Ms. Ufema to share some of her experiences and philosophies with us, and the following is an open letter from Joy Ufema to nursing students.

OPEN LETTER FROM A NURSE SPECIALIZING IN THE CARE OF THE DYING PATIENT

In nursing, we can always choose to avoid death; we simply go to the operating room, the newborn nursery, or some other area that is safe. Perhaps, in our own lives, we do not lose a parent, a child . . . someone we really love. But there will come a time in life when you will need some of the things that I am going to try to teach you in this letter—valuable things the dying have taught me. The time of that need is when you yourself die. Because 100 years from now, each of you and I will be nothing but a handful of dust.

First, it would be helpful to explore why we don't like death. Maybe the reasons are obvious because of the suffering we associate with death, because it is the end of living. In nursing, there is an additional reason. We have been taught, in past years, to be stoic, never divulging a diagnosis to a patient, never letting him tell we know either with our words (verbal behavior) or our emotions (nonverbal behavior). Perhaps, we are fearful of losing our professionalism. We simply go into a 20-year old leukemic's room, plunk down his tray and wisk ourselves right back out with a sigh of relief that we didn't say anything about his condition. Unfortunately, nurse, you did say it, nonverbally, by your very behavior.

We give off cues to the dying, and I try to make nurses aware of this. We send the message that we are uncomfortable in his presence, that we don't wish to remain in his room. Are we fearful that the patient will take us by the hand and ask, "I'm dying, aren't I?"

Another reason that we don't like death is that it reminds us of our own mortality. So, we give the patient a second cue: if you do know you are dying, I want you to act like you don't because that will make me more comfortable. I didn't want to be assigned to you three days in a row, it's not my fault I'm here . . . I really don't want to be here. Sure, I'll help give you good care for your treatments, bathe you, rinse your sore mouth, but please protect me from this. I don't want to think about it because I am only 20 years old, and I am not interested in dying or in any of the pain it takes to die. Well, maybe that's a new problem we have to face, nurse. Twenty-year-olds die; and so do ten-year-olds, . . . and so do two-year-olds.

I recognize these feelings because I have them, too, when I go to see a patient. I realize that I am just not going to get out of this world alive; on some days that's very scary to me.

I think we all have to start by being honest in dealing with our feelings about death. Once we have worked through them, we are better able to be honest and comfortable with our dying patients. This is the most important thing I can teach you. I can't give you the answers for every possible situation. Sometimes, when I go to see a patient, I don't even know what I am going to say.

And I think that is all right. In honesty, I simply tell the patient that I don't have the right words, but I assure him that I do care enough to stay with him. If he chooses to share his feelings with me, I will listen, and if he doesn't, that's okay, too; I will just stay by him. We cannot set criteria for someone else's death. Just because that person happens to be a patient in your hospital, and you happen to be assigned to him for that day, doesn't give you the right to set rules for him. Your comfort simply isn't as important as his. Remember, it's his turn now; eventually, it will be yours.

I place a tremendous importance on finding out from the patient what it is he wants. This can't be done by asking his mate, chaplain, doctor, or best friend. Only the patient can tell you what it is he wants, from whom he wants it and when. As I ask the patient this question, I am in a sense loading my guns for the coming fight, and I am loading them with the correct ammunition.

The following examples are true. The people I am writing about were my patients, beautiful people whom I loved, with whom I became emotionally involved, and with whom I cried.

Joan was a forty-two-year-old woman with carcinoma of the trachea. She had been in the hospital for about three weeks, going downhill very rapidly. One Saturday afternoon, her husband, who was probably traumatized by his wife's illness, had a minor automobile accident. I was called at home, out of my garden, by the hospital. Joan was hysterical and didn't believe any of the girls when they told her Harold was not seriously injured. The anxiety affected her breathing, and she was gasping for breath when I arrived.

You don't have to wear that lovely little white outfit to be a good nurse. In my Mickey Mouse T-shirt and wranglers, I ran to the hospital, simply grabbed an oxygen tank, attached Joan's lead to it and took her upstairs to see her husband. He was doing fine. Joan felt much better; I took her back to her room and settled her in for the night.

Harold had developed a few minor complications, and his physician decided that he should be hospitalized for a week or so. The same day I learned this news, Joan's roommate was discharged, and I came up with an idea that almost cost me my job. I suddenly thought that Joan might like to have her husband as a roommate. I asked her.

Gasping, she said, "Yes, could you do that, please?"

"Of course," I answered.

I went upstairs to see her husband. "Joanie would like to have you downstairs in her room. How do you feel about that?"

He loved the idea; it would be just fine, as he hoped to take Joan home to be there with him when the end came.

That settled it and I went to see the supervisor, cautiously, because, due to a shortage of beds, Joan was on a gynecology floor. The supervisor looked at me as if I had lost my mind: "A man on the GYN floor?—Absolutely not!"

I took a couple of deep breaths because I realized what the next step could cost me, and went to the head nurse. She was sympathetic but reacted negatively for a different reason.

She was concerned that Joan might die in her husband's presence.

That thought hadn't occurred to me, so I ran back upstairs to Harold. I was totally honest with him. Joan was critically ill; she could die very soon. He said that he knew what was coming but wanted to be with Joan anyway. "Joy,' he said, "let's do it."

Waiting for no one else's permission, I scrubbed Harold's bed, got him transferred down to the seventh floor, scrubbed the other bed and settled Joan and Harold into their own room. Both of them were beaming.

The nurses raised cain, temper tantrums trumpeted from nursing station to nursing station. My name was an anathema for a few weeks, and, for the first time, in my life I wasn't my usual ethical self. I lashed back at all, reminding them that Harold wasn't that great an imposition and couldn't they do something special for this patient who was dying? ... Couldn't they make it easier for her?

I looked in the following morning. Joan had slept twelve hours straight through, without analgesic or hypnotic. She had breakfasted with her husband and had kept the food down for the first time in three weeks. How do you know what to do? How do you know you are doing it right? You simply ask the patient what he wants, then you have the courage to follow through to help the person get it. If you don't care enough, if you ask flippantly, if you are not willing to follow through *all the way,* don't bother asking. I cared enough about Joan to risk my job, to risk everything to do what she needed when she needed it. And, this isn't necessarily the responsibility of the nurse to the patient. It is the responsibility of one human being to another. We do not always have our white dresses on. We are not always "the nurse," but we are always "the human being."

By the time you have reached this point in your text, you are probably well acquainted with the term "active listening," and I rated "listening" next to honesty in my contacts with dying patients. It really isn't something we should have to learn. We do it, almost by instinct, when we care. I did the right thing for Joan, but I also remember another time when I almost blew it.

Sometimes we do get tired and that is legitimate. I was working with Mr. Snipes, a patient who had a carcinoma of the lung. He had thrown several emboli and was bleeding badly, bringing a great flow of blood up through his mouth. I had changed his sheets three or four times that day—it was very hot and I was very tired, didn't have any lunch and wasn't *actively listening.* It was late and I wanted to get home. I had blood all over me and everything else. I finally got him cleaned up. Mr. Snipes took my hand, thanked me for the nursing care, and told me to take care of myself.

I was tired, not listening, said: "Okay, I will, bye." I sort of rushed to the door but when I got there it dawned on me; something inside of me had remembered to listen. I was slow to get it, but I did get it. I went back to his bed, took his hand and said: "You're saying good-bye, aren't you?"

He said that he was because he knew death was very near and that he wouldn't be there the next day. I thanked him for being my friend, for all he had taught me and told him how much I liked him. Then we said good-bye.

The next morning, as soon as I came on duty, I went to M-5. The bed was empty.

I was relating this story to a colleague, who commented that I would have felt like an awful fool if Mr. Snipes had been there when I went back the next day. Not at all. I would have rushed into his room and said, "You're still here and I'm so glad." We would have talked a little bit more; we would have had a little more time together. Nothing would have been lost. But so much would have been lost if some part of me were not listening, if I had not stopped at the door and gone back.

Sometimes, we'll look at a person and think, I can't tell whether to believe him or not. This is usually because his words are saying one thing and his behavior something else. We can all articulate a great deal that we don't feel, so it is usually the behavior that is believed. The words can be: I really care about you and I'll be back. But if you don't get back, it's your behavior (nonverbal message) that the patient is going to believe. Most of the time, it doesn't take a lot of words to tell the patient you really care. You tell him best by going directly to him as you enter his room, staying close to him, physically touching him, and asking him what his needs are. I'm sure you have all been taught about the little old lady who was lying in her bed, far down the hall; you enter the room to answer her light: What is it now, Mrs. Jones? "I want the bedpan." You just had the bedpan. "I know, but I need it again." Oh, all right. You give it to her, she tinkles a tiny bit, you abruptly rip it out from under her, slam-bang into the bathroom. You wash your hands but don't bother to give Mrs. Jones anything to wash her hands with and bustle out of the room. As you get to the door, she says: "Nurse." What now? "Could you please get me a drink of water?" Oh, all right. You plunk the pitcher down and don't think about holding the straw and that she's had a stroke and can't get her mouth set around it quite right. Meanwhile, you're tapping your toe, thinking of the 35 meds you have to pass, wishing she would hurry up. You start for the door again. "Nurse." Now what? "Could you fix the window blinds?"

What is she really saying? Verbally, she's asking for a bedpan, water, and adjustment of the light in her room. Nonverbally, she is saying, stay with me, please, I am frightened.

Often, the dying are saying this, too. But they are so neat, unless they are desperate, they won't impose on you because you have given all these cues that you can't handle it, or don't care. If you are uncomfortable, none of your words will work.

Once you become truly comfortable, the words are true and your behavior is true, both things click and then you are good. The dying check for cues. And, you get points if you sit on the patient's bed, if you look him in the eyes, if you touch him, if you are honest and come back when you say you will. This is your commitment when you want to give and when you want to care. It is all very simple and you don't have to work at it.

As you are learning from this textbook, I would want you all to repeatedly ask yourselves, who am I? and what am I good at? Do I want to be a nurse? What kind of a nurse do I want to be? What kind of a person do I want to be? Write down these questions and your answers and keep them in mind as you learn and grow. In this quest, discover what it is you do well and do it. Perhaps, like me, you will opt to work with dying patients, or you might have more to offer as a nurse in a gynecology clinic. Nursing has a place for us all, provided we find out what we do well, then do it well. Whatever direction you follow in your nursing career, maintain your integrity and the patient's dignity.

Joy Ufema, R.N.
Harrisburg Hospital
Harrisburg, Pennsylvania

7

Crisis Intervention

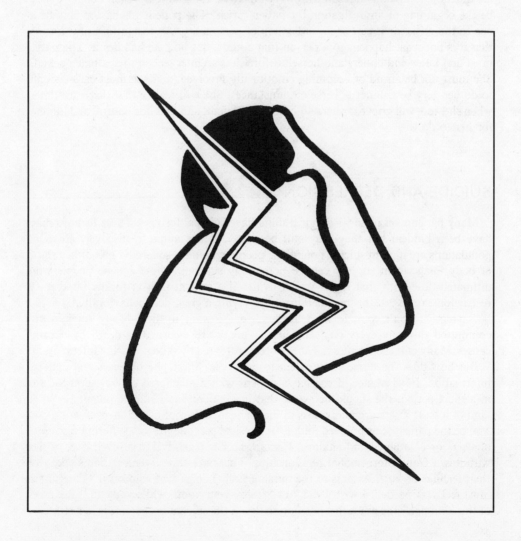

A dramatic change in one's life may be considered to be a crisis. A person's behavior in reacting to a crisis is really a symptom of the condition. Change is usually associated with the term "crisis." We all differ in our ability to tolerate crisis. We have varying levels of tolerance for adversity. What upsets one person may not upset another, but there are some crises that most people react to in a similar fashion, e.g., death, retirement, unexpected disability, hospitalization, etc. These are but a few.

Out-patients receive most of their crisis intervention from community resources. Potential suicide victims, in depression or loneliness, can call community hot lines instead of committing suicide. Many are helped, some are not. People with family, financial, or legal problems can be referred to community-based agencies for help.

Our main concern as nurses will be the hospitalized patient. Crises take place in the hospital arena on a daily basis. Often the patient's cry for help is said without words. The expression on the face of the newly hospitalized patient may be the nurse's only clue that all is not well. The patient may be experiencing a crisis because he fears unwanted diagnosis, or because he is reluctant to relinquish his privacy. Some patients are quiet on admission, and some are very talkative. In either case, their behavior may be the beginning of an evaluation for patient crisis. The patient's behavior may be a cue to the crisis, or it can be an indication of personality. An insightful nurse knows that it is not what happens to a person that counts, but how he handles it. The nurse must first know and understand herself before she can intervene in the patient's behalf. She must not be afraid of becoming emotionally involved, and she must care enough to do her very best under adverse circumstances. She will realize that there are times when she, too, will grieve for herself, or for her patient, and that it is natural and human for her to do this.

SUICIDE AND DEPRESSION

Many patients on medical–surgical units have suicidal feelings. These feelings may have been hidden, but they may still be there for the nurse to discover. Hospital populations are high in suicide potentials; people who have suffered a loss of health or of body image from surgery can be potentially suicidal. These can be people who ultimately lose faith that life is worth living. If a patient fails to follow his dietary restrictions, or to take his medications, he is saying a great deal behaviorally. He may be saying, "I don't want to be a burden," or "I want to die." Many suicides are committed this way every day, and just as many are recorded as death by natural causes. Many of these suicides may have been prevented by skilled nursing intervention.

But how does the nurse know when to intervene? First, she observes and collects information. For instance, if she has a patient who has suffered several severe losses in a short period, she should be aware that her patient has a suicide potential. What kind of losses? There are many: loss of independence, loss of health, loss of work, etc. Maybe the patient feels unloved, old, is in physical pain, depressed, suffering from loss of sleep, or is fatigued and anxious. Perhaps he has recently lost a loved one, or has withdrawn from interpersonal relationships. There are times when patients speak of their feelings of worthlessness to the nursing staff. The patient who says, "You nurses must feel very needed, I wish I did." or "Enjoy your youth while you can." Remarks of this kind place the nurse in a position to detect the suicide-prone. She is in a strategic position to intervene and save a life. There are reasons, however, why she may hesitate to intervene. She may feel that self-destruction is repugnant and refuse to recognize it in others. She may deny what she senses because she is threatened by it, or she may find that she is exhausted and depressed by her efforts to help, and she may dismiss her feelings with platitudes like, "I'm sure you will be feeling much better when you get home." Remarks like this cause the patient to withdraw. He will not reach out to her for help again. If a nurse has a gut reaction that her patient is feeling self-destructive, she should face the situation squarely and try to bring some of the patient's grieving process to the surface. She can do this by giving of herself and trying to understand just how her patient might be feeling. She knows that her patient has suffered several severe losses, so pat answers and remarks are not indicated. Pat answers create a defense for the nurse, which protects her from involvement. If she does not become involved, she can't help.

The patient will give hints and clues, many of them nonverbally, if the nurse will only look for them. The nurse should not fear open discussion about suicide, for if the patient feels that life is intolerable, talking about it will help him understand that he has the strength to work through his problems. Most patients have the resources to survive if they know that someone cares enough to help. Having someone care eases feelings of loneliness and depression. There are many people the nurse can consult with on behalf of the patient, so they can indicate they care, too, e.g., family and friends, neighbors, the physician, hospital volunteers, and people from community resources. Some community resources would be the psychologist, psychiatrist, social worker, and guidance counselor.

When a patient is depressed because he suffered losses, the intensity of his emotions can be reduced with the help of time, by talking it out, and with appropriate medication. The physician will order the medication, if the nurse will just consult with him, telling him how her patient is feeling and behaving. A quiet, comfortable interview with gentle questioning of the patient will show that you care about him, and that you recognize his calls for help. It will help him to realize that he is not alone and that his feelings are not so unusual. Sharing thoughts with the nurse may reduce the intensity of the patient's feelings. After a successful interview, the patient may say, "I feel better now; I've never talked this way with anyone before about this." When this happens, the nurse has truly intervened, and the patient's anxiety level has been reduced.

The nurse should not make any false promises to the patient. If she cannot deliver on a promise, trust will be destroyed, and a communication barrier will build between the patient and the nurse. When the interview has been completed, the nurse should make careful entries on the nursing care plan, so that the patient will have on-going follow-up. If possible, the same nurse should continue to visit and to care for the patient on a one-to-one basis. This will continue to assure him that he is cared for. The nurse can share what she has learned with the other team members, so that the nursing care plan will be meaningful for the patient. Further interviews can help build up his reasons for remaining alive and weaken his reasons for contemplating suicide. They can further draw out and use the patient's strengths.

The nurse who knows herself will be prepared to confront the issue of her own mortality when she deals with the suicide-prone patient. She knows that in order to understand the meaning of death, she must first understand the meaning of self. To be prepared to die is to understand what it would be to cease to exist as the selves we are. To know that is to know who and what we are. Without such knowledge, there can be no significant living. The nurse who has this understanding and philosophy can intervene therapeutically for her patients.

A life crisis for an individual can very well be hospitalization for the treatment of any acute illness. A stroke is but one example. Any hazardous event may be the beginning of a crisis, e.g., death, birth, or injury (physical or psychological). Many patients attempt to utilize old coping patterns in order to handle the new situation. The old patterns are unsuccessful and result in an acute psychological upset. The patient can resolve the crisis only when he learns to establish new coping patterns to deal with the new stress or loss. The nurse who knows this can help her patient apply new and specific coping patterns of behavior to the crisis. The nurse should help the patient identify the crisis and assist him in expressing his feelings about it.

If the patient has become withdrawn because his hospitalization is the crisis, it is beneficial if the nurse assists the patient with discussions that enable him to reenter his social world and regain some control over his environment.

CORONARY PATIENT GROUPS

Discussion groups comprised of patients may be an interventional approach for patients who have survived coronary attacks. Nursing staff are invited to attend and to participate. The groups meet at least three days a week and last for fifteen to thirty minutes. After each meeting the staff members meet and discuss the group's ability to relate and to socialize with one another. There should always be at least two staff members present at group meetings. Further discussion by the staff includes an assessment of the level of intervention. The patients in the group should be capable of some degree of verbal communication. Four patients in the group is an ideal composition. At meetings like this, the staff members utilize the opportunity to observe, and later discuss, the wealth of nonverbal communication that takes place. Expression on the faces of the group members, their gestures, or whether they fidget, smoke, tap their fingers and feet, and are restless are but a few of the meaningful observations that are made by the staff members. Some patients are very busy avoiding eye contact in these sessions. Some patients may seem weary and some depressed; some overtalk as a way to avoid real communication. It can be assumed that all of the patients share a fear of having had a coronary. Usually the patients are male, since more male than female patients have coronary attacks.

Coronary patients have a tendency to want to do more or less than they should. These sessions are a good way for them to discover just what level of physical activity is right. The staff members' participation can be valuable here, as they contribute the acceptable recommendations for appropriate activity. The patients can learn a great deal about their conditions as they begin to realize that they may build up a collateral circulation that will enable them to live a useful life and that it is not the end of living for them; they should be aware that they do not need to be so discouraged. Discussion with others also leads them to realize that they are not alone, that all is not lost, and that the crisis in their lives can be resolved.

As the group begins, the members first get acquainted. Then they start to learn about the different causes and effects of coronary attacks. At this time, the staff can remedy any misconceptions. Usually the patients begin to express their anxieties about the future. They may say, "How can I prevent another coronary?" "Will I have another one?" Sometimes they will talk about their plans for discharge in an unrealistic way. Staff members can gently point out obvious reality factors that are being ignored or overlooked. The staff members are there to be supportive and to clarify. This is how and when they intervene. They provide information regarding coronaries when asked, and they encourage the group members to express their concerns.

As the patients progress they start to trust one another and the staff, then their despair and feelings of helplessness surface; they discuss their anxieties. Some common concerns are the loss of control over their lives, and the fear of having another coronary. The thought of death is often a common theme in their discussions. Most patients are learning that their previous life-styles are now not practical; that they are adjusting to physical and social losses, that they are grieving over the loss of independence and the loss of body function. Often the patients become angry about their situations, and sometimes they displace their anger on the staff. They may blame themselves because they think they should be recovering faster. At this time, their anger and despair changes to realistic discussion about going home and the problems that exist there. Older patients worry about being a burden. Younger patients are concerned about the possibility of further sexual activity, employment, or job advancement. As more time elapses, the patients start to see their altered role in the family and in the community. The staff permits the patients to express their anger and frustration freely and helps them to identify ways of coping.

The last few meetings of the group often consist of providing trial weekend visits at home, or the actual discharge of the patient from the hospital. In all of the meetings, patients display feelings of apprehension, confusion, and ambivalence. As they near discharge, many of them fear that the staff has lost interest in them or that they are being rejected. These feelings are natural, and the staff makes this known to the patients. Some patients recall their memories of better days, when they felt successful. These feelings are good, because they help the patient be optimistic again, and they lead them to new feelings of self-esteem. They may not be able to be as active as they were in the past, but there are new ways to make a contribution to their society and community. The staff can help them to discover these.

Most patients agree finally that the group process helped them to tolerate their feelings of depression, and that it helped them to know what to expect in their futures regarding their illness and their ability to function. The group assisted them to learn that other patients had similar concerns and feelings about illness, hospitalization, and future. Within the group, each patient has the goal of independent functioning within his individual limits, and each patient is treated as an adult.

The nurses who participate as staff members learn a great deal about themselves and about their patients, so it is a learning experience for all involved. Throughout the entire group process, both nurses and patients may experience feelings of anxiety or depression and this is understandable, but there is an impact of security and acceptance for the patients as they learn to identify as a group. By being cohesive, they can express intense feelings and learn to trust. The supportive framework of the group benefits all involved. Some patients share their thoughts later with other patients during nongroup time, and many interact with their families when they visit. The group provides an opportunity for patients to react openly on their loss of function and their feelings about dependency and death.

Group meetings are also helpful for patients who are unable to verbalize. This can be seen by observing the changes in the expressions on their faces as time goes by. Their general attitudes and outlooks seem to be enhanced. Although these patients are not able to express themselves verbally, they see and hear others, and they realize that they are not alone. They can still understand others and can learn through others about themselves when they hear the patients who do verbalize. In this way they can see their own capabilities and limitations. There is no doubt that group meetings provide important insights into the responses patients make to a critical illness, and that they are good methods of crisis intervention. For the nurse who feels inexperienced in this element, there are many excellent courses available in group dynamics and nursing leadership.

Before the patient is discharged, he should be made aware of the community health centers that are available. These include centers such as walk-in psychiatric clinics, crisis-intervention units, suicide-prevention units, halfway houses, sheltered workshops, psychiatric units in general hospitals, group therapy, family therapy, and the mental health teaching that takes place in police stations, churches, outpatient departments, industries, and schools. If the patient becomes depressed or feels suicidal, he should get in touch with his physician. The physician can notify the nearest community mental health center and refer the patient there for further evaluation and group therapy. Private, individual therapy is another alternative. Many times the nurse will be the significant person in the life of the patient, and she is free to make an appropriate referral. For this reason, the nurse should also be familiar with the community health centers.

SUICIDAL PATIENTS _____

When self-destructive patients are hospitalized, they may have a positive response to hospitalization because someone is constantly with them. In these cases, the lethality of the home environment may not be fully appreciated, and the potential for suicide is high if the patients are pushed back into their suicidogenic environment. There may be an angry, rejecting, or exhausted partner in that environment. These patients may feel the rage and despair of the abandoned child when they go home. Once again, crisis intervention is the order of the day for the patient.

A suicidal patient may not be certain that he wants to die; nor is he convinced that he wants to live. This is the point where crisis intervention should occur. The nurse has the goal of developing a therapeutic environment to help build the patient's self-esteem by helping him to meet his emotional needs. She, in turn, needs the cooperation of other staff members and the physician so that a team approach can be established. As the nurse works closely with her patient, she helps him participate in social, recreational, or occupational activities. She seeks ways to reassure him that he is a worthwhile and useful human being. Emphasis should be placed upon applying safe opportunities for participation in the daily hospital routine. The nurse in crisis intervention cultivates the ability to be constantly aware of her patient's moods and his every activity.

Many authorities believe that all patients give a warning of their suicidal intentions either verbally or nonverbally. These warnings should be taken seriously. Such warning signals usually indicate the uselessness of life for that person. There is no real answer that applies to every situation. The method of dealing with the problem will vary with the situation and with the patient. Some suicidal patients merely make a gesture, others gamble that they will be stopped in time, and some are deliberate. Deliberate attempts indicate a plan for success at suicide. Those who gamble expect either success or failure of their attempt. Those who make a gesture hope that they will be intercepted during the attempt. All of the attempts are pleas for help, or pleas to be released from some unbearable or intolerable circumstance. Those who work in crisis intervention know that suicide attempts decrease when the patient feels secure and when there is a mutual trust between the patient and the nurse. This is why rapport with the patient is the most helpful prevention of suicide.

The loneliness of the long night is feared by many hospitalized patients. Facing a new day may be difficult for those patients who awaken in the early morning hours. Newly admitted patients should have a great deal of emotional support during the first few days. This will help them to accept their illness and hospitalization. During the period of hospitalization, the patient may have outside trauma caused by divorce or the serious illness and death of a loved one. This becomes an additional and severe loss for the patient who already has the trauma of hospitalization to cope with. The nurse will see this as an added complication to deal with.

The patient who is hostile because he is overwhelmed by discouragement should not be reacted to in the same way by the nursing personnel. This will only provoke the patient to become more angry, and a life may be lost because of it.

The attitude of acceptance by the nurse toward her patient can be communicated nonverbally, as well as verbally. Instead of chastisement, there should be loving empathy. This support helps to put the patient at ease. It makes him feel that he is understood. Caring and concern by the nurse make the patient feel that he is worthy and loved. Suicidal patients are highly troubled and sensitive people, and they can sense an unfeeling attitude of the nurse very easily. The nurse should remember that her patients are able to sense her attitude of acceptance or rejection without words. Just as the nurse searches for nonverbal communication from her patient, she should remember that her patient is always receiving nonverbally from her. Things will go well if the nurse pays attention to what her patient is saying and feeling; she should be a responsive listener. In order to do this, she listens between the lines that the patient expresses. She notes how he acts, how interested he is in eating, how his moods change, whether he seems agitated, how he sleeps, whether he is impulsive, and how he faces his feelings of loss. All of this nonverbal information can be valuable.

When patients lose all hope of having a meaningful future, it is a good time to suggest alternatives. These alternatives must be realistic and must be conveyed honestly and gently. The patient has to be convinced that he can be optimistic in spite of his problems. When he has greater insight into his feelings of despair, they lessen. This is what intervention is all about. The patient begins learning to identify his problem, and along the way learns to develop insight and understanding that enable him to cope with these problems. Through this method, he moves from negative feelings to a positive outlook and crisis intervention has been successful.

The patient's sense of isolation has diminished, and he is able to be involved with others in humanistic ways. The emergency of the crisis is only concluded when he is able to be at home concerned with the attitude that he wants to live and is free from feelings of anger and depression.

THE GRIEVING PROCESS _____

There are many reasons why patients grieve because of a loss: unfamiliar surroundings of the hospital, the hospital experience itself, the change of body image that results from aging or surgery, an abortion, the illness of a friend or a relative, divorce, the loss of employment while hospitalized, or having to give up a life's dream because of a resulting handicap. The perceptive nurse asks herself, "Why does my patient hurt?" "How can I help my patient put the pieces together again?" She knows that the level of stress has built up beyond her patient's level of tolerance and that her patient is in crisis. Of all the roles that a nurse must assume, none requires more skill than helping patients cope with their grieving process. When hospitalized, the patient may find that his usual ways of coping with stress and anxiety are not available to him. He feels vulnerable. His task is to learn new coping skills, and this is what the nurse is there to help him do. She is there to help him restore his psychological equilibrium. To do this, she makes use of all the possible social network of people who are important to the patient. Sometimes there are not any or enough significant others in the patient's life. This may well be what his crisis is all about. If it is, the nurse has her work laid out for her. She will have to find ways to help her patient feel strengthened. She will try to convince him that he is worthy and strong enough to tolerate his adversity; that this is an alternative to resolving his dilemma. Her therapy should focus on the immediate problem that the patient is facing. If she can involve others, she can gradually assume a less active role. In some instances, this intervention can be done in two sessions with the patient. If the nurse finds that it is safe to leave the situation but that continued help is indicated, she will then assist in the referral process as mentioned previously. Grieving is something that everyone must deal with sometime during his life. Those who manage to grieve successfully may resume their lives and become stronger than they were before. The nurse should tell the patient about this possibility, since it is honest and realistic.

There was a case where a 16-year-old male patient lost his mother while he was in the hospital. The relatives, who were afraid to interfere with his health, did not tell him until it was time for discharge from the hospital. Three weeks later, he returned home only to discover his loss and to find that his relatives had pretty well finished their grieving process. He was alone because there was no one to help him with his grief. He became physically ill again and had to return to the hospital. By this time, he was in crisis, and the nurse who knew this history could focus on the immediate problem that her patient was facing. It is not always this easy when it comes to assessing and to identifying the problem, since no two situations are the same.

There are times when others fail to recognize the loss the patient feels. Take the young female patient who has just had an undesired medically prescribed abortion. She was hospitalized, in strange surroundings, and away from relatives and friends. This prevented her from grieving, for it seemed to her that others were not concerned about her loss. Since hospital personnel are used to abortions, she felt that hers was of little consequence to them. No one seemed to want to pay attention to her feelings until an empathetic nurse one day sensed her patient's mood and inquired. The patient fortunately grieved and talked about her feelings before she went home. This was a good thing because this woman may very well have been one of the many women who present themselves to psychiatric clinics later, when it is harder to resolve a crisis. The shorter the crisis, the less the prolonged trauma. In this case, the nurse was able to discover that her patient was blaming herself for the loss of her baby. The nurse was able to assure her that she was not at fault, that all had been done that could be done, and that life had many good things to offer her yet. It is helpful for people to talk about their turmoil because it relieves the burden they feel inside. This case is a classic example of this truism. It should be noted that the nurse picked up the patient's feelings nonverbally. The patient's mood and facial expression were the clues for the nurse. The fact that the nurse was a perceptive, caring person made the crisis intervention possible.

In another instance, there was a 15-year-old girl who died of an overdose of heroin. The parents appeared to be stoic as they sat outside of the emergency room. They seemed to be maintaining a self-imposed image—the image that it really did not matter so much—and that they were strong. The emergency room nurse sensed that they were not able to grieve. She stopped by them and merely put a hand on each parent's shoulder. She stood silently with them. Suddenly, the father cried, and the mother followed with sobs. The grieving process was taking place. The nurse had truly intervened in a crisis, and she had done it without any words. Words did evolve as the parents unburdened their feelings of guilt and loss.

A Search For Meaning

The following section relates to Dr. Viktor E. Frankl's profound work, *Man's Search for Meaning: An Introduction to Logotherapy,* [16] in which the author, a psychiatrist, describes his experiences as a longtime prisoner in German concentration camps during the Second World War. Frankl refers to the other inmates as patients, because from the moment of their internment, they needed care.

After being stripped of his own identity, after the indignity of being reduced to his naked self, Dr. Frankl discovered that there was still a meaning to living. Having watched many men die as a result of neglect and deprivation, under the most inhuman conditions, there was also a meaning to dying. If a man transcended such humilities, he could still live or die with dignity. As long as man clings to his own very personal meanings for being and existing, there can be meaning for him in suffering. This positive outlook enables him to tolerate and to endure anything and everything that happens to him.

Each man's meaning is his own, within him to discover. This process is private and usually nonverbal in nature. It strengthens him regardless of how weak his body may be. It enables him to achieve in his suffering. The patients in concentration camps who were able to do this survived.

> The thought of suicide was entertained by nearly everyone, if only for a brief time. It was born of the hopelessness of the situation, the constant danger of death looming over us daily and hourly, and the closeness of the deaths suffered by many of the others.

What were some of the meanings of these patients, and why did they not commit suicide? "In one life there is love for one's children to tie to; in another life, a talent to be used; in a third, perhaps only lingering memories worth preserving. To weave these slender threads of a broken life into a firm pattern of meaning and responsibility" was the object and challenge of these patients who wanted to survive.

> Swiftly, too, come strategies to preserve the remnants of one's life, though the chances of

surviving are slight. Hunger, humiliation, fear and deep anger at injustice are rendered tolerable by closely guarded images of beloved persons, by religion, by a grim sense of humor, and even by glimpses of the healing beauties of nature—a tree or a sunset. . . . But these moments of comfort do not establish the will to live unless they help the patient make larger sense out of his apparently senseless suffering.

The patients who were able to do this learned that "to live is to suffer, to survive is to find meaning in the suffering. If there is a purpose in life at all, there must be a purpose in suffering and in dying. But no man can tell another what this purpose is," for it is nonverbal. "Each must find out for himself, and must accept the responsibility that his answer prescribes. If he succeeds, he will continue to grow in spite of all indignities." Frankl is fond of quoting Nietzsche: "He who has a *why* to live can bear with almost any *how*." For our purposes, this means that once our patient wants to live, when he discovers his meaning for living, he will naturally set about determining how to do it.

When "all the familiar goals in life are snatched away, what alone remains is the last of human freedoms—the ability to choose one's attitude in a given set of circumstances. The patients were only average men, but some at least, by choosing to be worthy of their suffering, proved man's capacity to rise above his outward fate."

As a prisoner, Viktor Frankl attempted to hang on to his whole former life when he tried to preserve his scientific manuscript, which was his life's work. This was discarded as worthless by guards, just as all other possessions were torn from patients to be used or destroyed by ruthless others. Frankl made an effort to recall his manuscript in bits and pieces throughout his imprisonment. His manuscript had meaning for him; it related to his thoughts of a future, it was something to cling to, and it helped him maintain his sanity and survive.

At critical moments in a naked existence, Frankl believes he survived because of some strange sensations. There was the grim sense of humor and a strange kind of cold curiosity about surviving. He feels that these sensations seemed to protect his state of mind.

How can nurses engaged in crisis intervention benefit from Dr. Frankl's experiences? They have learned to fortify their patients as well as themselves, for they know that the patient who feels self-destructive because of despair can be helped to discover his meaning for living, and that the patient who has an incurable illness can be helped to discover his meaning for suffering and dying.

The nurse can gently ask the patient, "What has meaning for you? When the patient begins to think in this direction, he starts to transcend his crisis. He chooses to be worthy of his suffering and lives.

Frankl believes that "tears may indicate that man has the greatest of courage, the courage to suffer." This could be reassuring for the nurse who is consoling her patient who is in crisis. She can say, "Don't be afraid to cry; it may be helping you to cope. You are so courageous." Tears often open the first door to real communication, and they are nonverbal.

If patients who feel hopeless can be helped to look toward the future, they are in a better position to cope with their crisis. The nurse can help the patient achieve this status by employing a number of nonverbal methods. For example, she can make an appointment for her patient, who has an order for physical therapy. She can make the appointment for tomorrow or next week. When she does this she has told the patient, without any words, that "We want and expect you to be alive. We have a place for you in the future."

Another positive nonverbal gesture aimed at the future is to provide the patient with a weekly schedule of his hospital routine or activities. This serves as evidence that he is very much a part of the future.

Viktor Frankl's views focus on the meaning of human existence, as well as on man's search for such a meaning. According to him, "the striving to find a meaning in one's life is the primary motivational force in man." If those in nursing and medicine believe this, they will serve their patients in crisis well and help them discover a meaning for existence.

It should be noted that, as Frankl cared for many ill or dying patients, he did so with a wealth of nonverbal communication. He gently touched their hands, soothed their fevered brows, and wept with them. Perhaps we in nursing can do this for our patients.

8

Sexual Behaviors

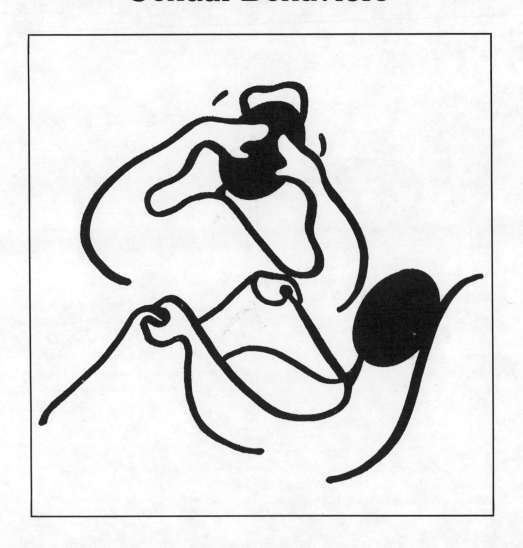

We are probably more sophisticated and enlightened about sex, today, than ever before in our history. But sexual acting out, in the hospital environment, still causes problems. Essentially, behavior that is overtly sexual on the part of one person can be threatening to another. Unsolicited sexual behavior is often viewed as an invasion of the private rights and person of an individual. In some social settings, we see examples of this as a man tries to physically draw away from a woman who has attached herself, without invitation, to his arm—or, when a woman angrily pushes aside the hand of a man whose behavior has become intimate. During most social contacts, however, people do observe spatial distance. They do not invade each other's private space. In the hospital environment, by necessity, there is a narrowing of that social distance, mainly because intimate care is rendered by one person (nurse) to another (patient).

Patients do not arrive at the hospital in a sexual void. They bring their individual sexuality with them, just as they bring their other basic human needs. Occasionally, patients experience sexual excitement from an intimate care procedure.

Many nursing students are afraid this will happen during a procedure and worry that they will not be able to act professionally if it does. They fear that they will not be able to look at the patient, continue speaking to him, or that they might blush, giggle, or in some other way transmit nonverbally their embarrassment and confusion. In most cases, the patient is just as confused and as embarrassed by the accidental arousal. With experience and conditioning, nurses usually worry less as they come to realize that the patient's reaction is normal, relatively common, and in no way aberrant.

There are some people who see nurses as poorly equipped to deal with sexual behaviors. This is, perhaps, in part, due to our reluctance to do so in the past. Because of the concept of total nursing care, many nurses today are more involved in humanistic aspects than they were a few decades ago. Sex, as a basic human need, is taught in some nursing curricula, and probably should be included in curricula for all levels of nursing. When nurses learn to view sexual needs in the same terms as other human needs, they will be better prepared to deal with sexual incidents.

An inexperienced nurse who has not had some education in human sexuality might find herself over-reacting to a patient's suggestive comments. Nonverbally, her embarrassment or anger would be communicated to the patient. Blushing or tears would tell him that she was flustered. By abruptly pulling back and away from the patient or by a firm stare, she would telegraph her anger.

The patient may react to the nurse's nonverbal behavior with more aggressive behavior, or he may himself become embarrassed or angry. The nurse can be very disturbed over situations like the one illustrated. She may be afraid to enter the patient's room again, or she may seriously question her own competency. Incidents of a sexual nature can be managed in a manner that will not interfere with the basic nurse–patient relationship. Admittedly, it is not always easy to develop the insight and the skills that make this possible. This is especially true since many nurses have not been prepared, as a part of their education, to deal with patients in sexual matters. The picture is further complicated by the fact that there is no guide for measuring their own competency in these matters.

The consideration of sex in the nurse–patient relationship is easier to manage when we start with one basic principle and proceed. There is no valid criterion for evaluating the sexual needs of any individual or group of individuals. If sexual needs cannot be evaluated, sexual needs cannot be judged.

When a nurse judges a patient's sexual behavior, the possibility for therapeutic interaction is greatly reduced. Judgments are not confined to the behavior only, as they can encompass feelings about when the behavior is enacted and who is involved.

For instance, a nurse may feel that she has no negative feelings on the subject of masturbation. Her perception of her own attitude is reinforced when she happens to notice a two-year-old masturbating, and thinks to herself: "That's quite all right, most infants do it, he's just a baby." However, she might have to examine her attitude when, upon entering a patient's room unexpectedly, she observes a seventy-year-old woman in the act of masturbation, and feels disgust and revulsion toward the patient. If the case of the seventy-year-old evokes strong feelings in the nurse, her relationship with the patient might become deleterious. Yet, biologically, there is no difference between the two cases. The two-year-old and the seventy-year-old were both gratifying a sexual need. The difference was only in the eyes of the observing nurse. Masturbation by the two-year-old did not disgust the nurse. Perhaps, she had been exposed to such child development authorities as George L. Engel,[17] who wrote that, "In some children, as early as the second year, and in most children in the third and fourth years, there is an increasing awareness of the pleasurable sensation from the genitals. Casual fingering of and playing with the genitals and actual masturbatory activity may begin within the first year. . . ." Awareness that the child's act was natural and normal allowed the nurse, cited in this case, to accept the behavior without anger or discomfort. People were not always so enlightened. No too many decades ago, some young children discovered in the act of masturbation had their hands put into restraints.

This nurse, apparently, had difficulty with her attitude toward the seventy-year-old patient whom she observed in the act of masturbation. Her feelings may have been based on the incorrect assumption that older people do not have sexual needs, or embarrassment in seeing the behavior in a mature person of her own sex. The nurse might have, with more understanding, come to accept the latter incident, just as her colleagues of some years ago came to accept the first. Readings and courses in the area of gerontology, with emphasis on the biological needs of the elderly may have provided her with more insight, thereby helping her to form a new attitude.

Sexual Attitudes

Attitudes, as discussed earlier in this work, are feelings that affect our behavior. Referring again to the illustration, the nurse observed the patient in a behavior that caused her to have certain feelings; those feelings became part of her attitude, which in turn affected her behavior. Let us assume that the nurse recognized her own negative feelings, determined not to let them block her nursing of the patient, concentrated on the delivery of good care and, purposefully, always spoke politely to the patient. It would work—almost. The patient would certainly pick up on the nurse's nonverbal cues expressed in the distance between nurse and herself during verbal exchanges, the rapid pace of procedures, or the lack of extra time and caring. The patient might feel that the nurse did not like her or was trying to punish her for something.

If the patient realized that the nurse had seen her in the act of masturbating, she might view the nurse's attitude—apparent in nonverbal cues—as punitive. Nonverbal behavior can be just as punitive as any spoken word.

There are times when the nurse's attitude causes her to think there is something sexual in a patient's behavior when there is not. A night nurse, for example, in going off duty reported that Mr. W. was exposing himself and that he had done so many times during her shift. The patient, a sixty-nine-year-old male, was diagnosed as having a urinary dysfunction. He was an immigrant from Eastern Europe, and his spoken English was not fluent. The night nurse reported that she constantly pulled the bed clothes back over the patient and finally reprimanded him, saying that the hospital simply did not tolerate *that kind* of behavior.

When the day nurse arrived to render care, she observed that the patient was restless. His palms were moist, and he appeared tense and apprehensive. He glared angrily as the day nurse approached, saying nonverbally all that he was unable to verbalize in English. The day nurse was not intimidated by his behavior and decided to inspect the genital area. She treated the patient very professionally, saying, "Let me see if I can make you more comfortable." The patient did not understand and remained anxious. The nurse continued to speak softly although she realized the patient was not following her words; she smiled, gestured, and tried to indicate that she wished to help him. Finally, the patient began to understand and relaxed a little. As the nurse examined the patient, she discovered that the indwelling catheter was taut, squeezed between the metal portion of the bed and the side rail, creating a condition that caused the patient discomfort. The nurse released the tension on the catheter, alleviating the patient's pain.

There were no more incidents with the patient's bed clothes. Because of his inability to verbalize, the patient may have been trying to indicate his distress to the night nurse, who, in turn, saw the behavior out of context. She did not consider complications with the catheter but saw the presenting behavior only in terms of a male patient exposing his genital area.

Feelings toward another person's sexuality can exist in cases where no overt behavior is present. Some of the areas that are occasionally difficult for people to handle attitudinally are: changes in sex from male to female or female to male, male and female impersonation, and treatments of a sexual nature that are basically cosmetic. Not too many years ago, anyone interested in changing his or her sex had to sneak away to some remote facility in Europe. Things are different today. Many sex-change procedures and surgeries are carried out in our most prestigious hospitals. Despite the general change in feeling, patients who are hospitalized for treatment that involves their sexual identity or sexual self-image are apt to be especially sensitive to both verbal and nonverbal behavior. They may consciously look for cues in the nurse's behavior that tell how she is really feeling about them.

A female patient who had been hospitalized for a mammoplasty to increase the size of her breasts related the following incident.

Most of the nurses were nice, but there was this one who really got to me. It wasn't that she did anything wrong. She was always polite, sort of crisply efficient, if you know what I mean. But I just sensed that she thought I was doing something wrong. When taking my pulse, she held my wrist like it was a hot potato, and she always spoke to me from across the room or from the doorway, never up close where our eyes could meet. One day, I just lost control when she came in and screamed at her that it was none of her business what I did with my own breasts. I felt terribly bad about what I did and apologized later. She must have really thought I was nuts, but then I guess she did from the beginning.

Attitudes that are judgmental do block communication, and those attitudes do not have to be verbalized to be damaging. The nurse in this illustration must have been very surprised by the patient's outburst, since her nursing competency and verbal behavior had been above reproach. Perhaps, she was not even aware that she was sending nonverbal messages of disapproval. If the nurse had been aware that her feelings were getting through to the patient, she might have been able to work through them to create a more therapeutic environment.

However, there are occasions when rapport between patient and nurse cannot be established within the allotted time of the hospitalization. The problem can be due to the nurse's attitude toward the patient or to the patient's attitude toward the nurse. This situation is to be expected from time to time, since no one person can successfully interact with all people. When this situation does occur, it is generally a wise policy for the nurse to advise her supervisor, requesting that someone else be assigned to the patient. As long as these circumstances are relatively infrequent, the nurse should not feel that her professional competency is in question.

Acting Out Sexually

There are many situations involving sex; some such as masturbation and fantasy, generally, do not involve the nurse personally. She is not physically involved in the patient's acting out. But other incidents of acting out do involve the nurse, and the occurrences are frequent for both male and female nurses. So far, we have presented this book, for the most part, in terms of the male patient and the female nurse solely for the purpose of clarification in illustrative dialogues and narratives. We do recognize the important role of men in nursing and are cognizant that patients act out sexually with male nurses as readily as they do with female nurses.

In our society, female patients probably have more ways to act out sexually than do male patients. The female patient can have her hair done, apply make-up, don her prettiest negligee, and behave in a physically seductive manner with male physicians and male nurses. A young male nurse told of a female patient, hospitalized for a fractured femur, who constantly rang while he was on duty. She complained of phantom lumps in her breast and would ask the nurse to see if he could feel the lumps. This request was always accompanied by many comments about her own loveliness and sexual desirability.

Female nurses have similar encounters as with the male patient who rubs against them during a procedure, or puts his arm around their hips. The patient may do his acting out verbally, suggesting a mutual sexual activity, commenting on the nurse's anatomy, or speculating on her personal sex life.

When the patient involves the nurse in a sexual situation—whether the behavior is verbal or physical—the nurse should deal with the presenting behavior immediately. It is going to be easier to manage the subsequent interaction if she remains nonjudgmental and deals only with the behavior. Comments such as: "How dare you" . . . "What do you think I am" . . . are neither effective nor professional responses because they convey disapproval of the patient's sexuality and rejection. The same negative feelings are communicated just as efficiently nonverbally by such behaviors as abrupt withdrawal from the patient's room, scowling, or tense body posture. Instead, the nurse should tell the patient that she realizes he has his needs and those needs are normal, but that it is not appropriate for him to express them to her. The reason that the behavior is inappropriate is that the nurse's exclusive role is to help the patient get well.

She is directed toward meeting the nurse care goal, and she does not want behavior, either his or hers, geared to anything except reaching that goal. The nurse should be rather assertive as she discusses the problem with the patient. She should emphasize that the behavior is inappropriate only in terms of the nurse–patient relationship, but that it is not inappropriate human behavior.

It would be impossible to present words or phrases that could be used by all nurses in all situations. The words will be your own, but they should convey your meaning clearly to the patient. The principle is that sexual behavior is evaluated only in terms of its appropriateness to the nursing situation. This should not vary and may be used by nurses, both male and female, in heterosexual incidents—and, in homosexual incidents.

An interaction consists of verbal and nonverbal dynamics. The focus of an interaction that deals with any form of sexual acting out should be on the behavior that is a manifestation of the patient's sexual needs. If the patient were to reach for a glass of water because he was thirsty, the nurse would assist him with the glass, unless water were contraindicated; in such cases, she would explain why it is not possible for him to have water at this time and advise him when it would again be available to him. She would not respond in a punitive manner to the patient's need for water, any more than she would be punitive of his nutritional or eliminative needs. Sex is a recognized biological necessity, and nurses should approach it as such even when the presenting behavior is in a context that is personally unfamiliar or uncomfortable.

Long-term patients may have different sexual needs than short-term patients. For instance, a patient hospitalized for hand and arm burns may begin to show some signs of sexual frustration as his hospitalization lengthens. It is not always easy to totally accommodate the patient's sexual needs within the hospital environment, but there are some ways that the nurse can help the patient to cope with his feelings. She can, for example, ask the patient if he is feeling some need for privacy, state that she would be glad to close the door (or put up a screen) for awhile. She might add that she would advise the staff that the patient wanted some time to himself, that he would ring when he was ready to have the door opened again. She should, whenever possible, extend the same accommodation when the patient's significant other is visiting.

Sex, like communication, is two way. Nurses are as capable of acting out sexually as patients are. Professionally, however, most nurses do not, because consciously seductive behavior would be unethical. Still, patients do, on occasion, see the nurse as flirtatious or seductive. The patient's perception can be based on his own faulty interpretation of the nurse's behavior, or on behavior that the nurse is not fully aware of. The nurse who is having problems in this area should become more aware of her own behaviors, especially her nonverbal cues and make adjustments when they are indicated.

Sometimes, the nurse and patient are mutually attracted to each other. When this happens, the nurse still has a professional role to fill. She must meet the health needs of the patient and cannot, as a professional person, engage in anything that would be deleterious to the patient's health goal. There is, undoubtedly, a great deal of controversy over how this situation should be handled. The consensus from a sampling of nurses, ranging from Master's level to one- and two-year graduates, who were asked this question, seems to indicate that many nurses feel the best approach is to tell the patient that you are also attracted to him and would like to see him again when you are no longer his nurse.

Altered Sexual Self-Image

Patients who have undergone medically indicated surgeries or treatments that affect their sexual functioning or sexual self-image require special understanding. Physical pain can be eased by medication, but the patient's psychological pain may be more devastating and more difficult to relieve. The nurse's manner of care delivery will be as important as the care itself. The patients will be especially sensitive to the nurse's nonverbal behavior and very quick to pick up on any negative cues. Intimate care procedures may be particularly difficult for the patient who will gauge the time the nurse spends on the procedure. If the nurse appears to rush, the patient may read into her behavior an indication of revulsion and think she wants to be away from him as soon as possible, or that it disgusts her to touch him. Procedures should be done slowly and gently; the nurse should indicate that she has all the time the patient needs; eye contact should be established and maintained; the nurse should touch the patient's hand or arm whenever appropriate; back rubs should be long and soothing. By touch contacts, the nurse is telling the patient that his altered body is all right. As she continues to show no aversion to the patient, he may come to realize that other people will also accept him. This realization can be the patient's first step toward adjustment and rehabilitation.

The nurse who applies humanistic principles to her own delivery of care does, on occasion, run the risk of becoming overly involved with the patient. Caring is a basic component of nursing and only becomes detrimental when the nurse's feelings interfere with her primary function. A male nurse had difficulty with his own feelings when he was assigned a thirty-year-old male patient who had undergone an orchidectomy for the removal of both testicles. Nurse and patient were the same age and shared many common interests. The patient was responding to the surgery with extreme depression and exhibited suicidal behavior. He shared his feelings with the nurse saying, "I'd rather be dead than to continue living this way."

The nurse later reported that he was unable to say anything to the patient because he saw himself in the patient's position and could only wonder what his own response might be. He discussed his concern at several staffing meetings and began to realize that he was relating too closely to the patient's condition. He was feeling pity rather than empathy. The nurse began to work through his own feelings; he reassessed the care plans and the nursing goals for the patient, and he began to look for ways to increase the patient's self-image. In discussing the case later the nurse said, "I really used nonverbal techniques with the patient. He didn't seem to want to talk about it, and I didn't feel I should force the conversation. Through my actions, I tried to let him know that I saw him as a man and a valuable person."

Situations involving individual sexuality or sexual acting out require a sensitive and humanistic approach. Nurses will manage sexual subjects more humanistically if they are cognizant of basic human needs and remember to address only the appropriateness of the presenting behavior. Initial awkwardness does not indicate any lack of competency. Perhaps the first time the nurse administered oxygen, she also felt some insecurities, but, with time, the procedure became smoother.

9
Some Nursing Dynamics:
Past and Present

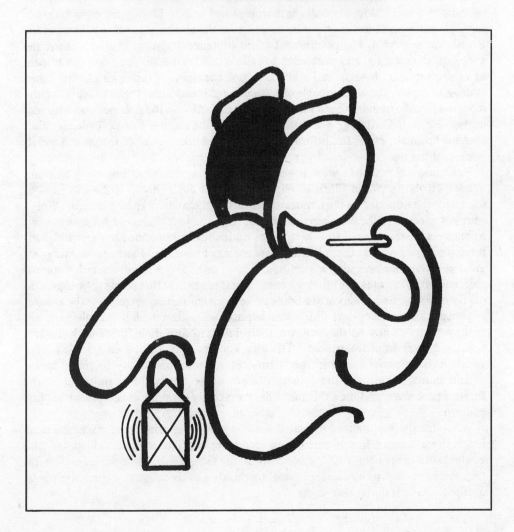

Most people are familiar with the name Florence Nightingale. Many people seem to identify her as the ideal of all the best that was and is in nursing.

In a sample questioning of nurses, nursing students and former patients who were asked to identify Florence Nightingale, only a handful were familiar with the biography of the first lady of nursing. But everyone questioned did have a very clear concept of who Florence Nightingale was symbolically. Nursing personnel generally viewed her as: (1) the first nurse to have the insight to recognize the need for organization in nursing; (2) an innovator who realized that a designated group should be trained to care for the sick and the wounded; (3) the originator of the concept of bedside care; and (4) the one who set the precedent for our own nursing tradition. Former patients saw Florence Nightingale as: (1) a model, an ideal that all nurses should be or should strive to achieve; (2) a very good and unselfish person; (3) someone who was willing to help all people with all their needs—spiritual and emotional, as well as medical.

Historically, Florence Nightingale was born in 1820 and died in 1910. She was a nursing pioneer and hospital reformer. Early in life she became interested in hospital work and studied methods of hospital administration through Europe. Eventually, she established a hospital for English gentlewomen in London. During the early stages of the Crimean War, there was a public uproar over the terrible state of treatment of the British war wounded. The government asked Florence Nightingale to reorganize the hospitals; she accepted and proceeded to raise a band of nurses and travel with them to a British military hospital in Turkey. She took command of the hospital, established systems to replace the indescribable chaos and, in this endeavor, began to lay down the modern scientific foundations of nursing. She consulted with the American government during our own Civil War and with the French during the Franco-Prussian War, founded hospitals, raised funds for medical care, and became one of the most honored women of her age.

Her name still embodies what is generally viewed as the finest in nursing care and nursing attributes. When Florence Nightingale went out at night, lantern in hand to search for the wounded on the Crimean battlefields, the soldiers knew she cared. Words were not necessary. She was there looking for them, helping them, not because she had to but because she wanted to. The soldiers undoubtedly responded to her with gratitude, appreciation, and affection. That response must have been Florence Nightingale's greatest reward for accepting a hard and difficult task, and it is still the one unspendable, unbankable, untaxable nursing benefit. But it is a benefit that seems to be diminishing for many nurses in many areas. Some professional nurses no longer have the amount of patient care that they once did. Administrative tasks keep them in the office and out of the patients' rooms. As they improve their skills and education, they find themselves promoted away from the patients. Teaching and consulting draw nurses away from patient areas. Specialization further limits the nurse's opportunity to relate to her patient humanistically, as the operating room nurse observes him only during the surgical procedure, and the CCU nurse must make his life support equipment her first concern.

While for the hospitalized patient the nurse is still the prime care-giver, she is no longer the sole care deliverer. There is an abundance of skilled and semiskilled staff who interact with the patient: EKG technicians, X-ray technicians, lab technicians, respiratory therapists and technicians, physical therapists and technicians, speech therapists, occupational therapists, and so on.

A newly admitted patient may see the professional nurse at the tail end of a long parade of staff. A lab technician draws the patient's blood and collects the urine specimen. An aide or a volunteer wheels the patient to his room. If an EKG is indicated, it is done by an EKG technician. An aide generally does the surgical "prep" and administers the enema when one is required. The patient's first contact with the nurse may not be until the evening medications are disbursed. At this point, no nurse/patient relationship has been established. The patient who is unhappy with his treatment or nervous about his hospitalization may vent his anger. The nurse will be his most likely target. He will hold her responsible for the way he has been treated. The nurse who does not have a good grip on her own emotions and an insightful approach to patient care may respond with equal negativism. She feels that she has been singled out for blame that belongs to others; her shift has been long and exhausting and she neither needs nor appreciates the patient's hostility. So she, in turn, mentally notes that the patient in 302 is difficult and may even compound her original error by sharing that information with other staff members. And the misunderstanding spreads. The morning nurse notices the light above 302 and thinks: Oh, that one is at his bell again. Perhaps it is the first time that the patient's bell has been on. She should answer the call and upon entering the patient's room, politely say something like: "Yes, Mr. Jones, what can I do for you?"

But if her tone, her posture, and her facial expression are saying: "Now what?" The patient reads the nonverbal message and an impasse is very quickly reached. The patient is labeled difficult; the nurses may appear indifferent, callous, or cold. It does happen; we have all seen it happen. If the nursing procedures are good, if the hospitalization is successfully terminated, and if the stay is brief, patient and nurse go their separate ways after a mutually unrewarding experience. The patient's overt or covert hostility may remain for a time. Perhaps he will write a letter to the hospital administrator complaining of poor nursing care, or insist to his physician that he will never allow himself to be admitted to that hospital again, or see an attorney about some minor or imagined infraction of accepted nursing procedure; or the patient may merely shake his head sadly and think to himself: "If Florence Nightingale knew what nurses were like today, she would turn over in her grave."

It is a great waste when this happens, because most patients are not difficult. They are simply reacting to a new, often frightening, environment. Nurses are not indifferent, callous, or cold; most are reacting to the pressures of time and priority. They are, generally, sincerely interested in their patients' welfare, although many have not mastered the skill of communicating that concern to the patient, especially on nonverbal levels.

THE GOOD PATIENT CONCEPT _____

In nursing, we speak of concepts. There is, for example, the positive concept of total patient care. But there is also a negative concept that blocks therapeutic nurse/patient relationships: the concept of the good patient. The concept in itself is not detrimental. If we see the patient as someone who is recuperating in accordance with medically sound expectations, the concept is not therapeutically unsound. But when we set goals and objectives for the patient, we have to consider that patient's background. What has the patient experienced prior to coming to the hospital, and what will happen to him when he returns home to complete his recuperation? We can look at the appendectomy patient and set goals that, at the end of a certain period of time, the patient will be able to get out of bed, ambulate in the halls, and do a self-bath. What we do not realize when we set these goals is that we are, generally, totally unaware of what is going on in that patient's life. There may be an angry, hostile mate at home who is upset over the cost of the patient's hospitalization, or undone household chores. The patient can be deeply stressed over family or financial matters, and his hospitalization may be yet another link in a chain of crises that has brought him to the end of his coping capabilities. We do not, unfortunately, always consider all the environmental, social, and emotional dynamics of the patient's situation and are, therefore, inclined to run out of patience with the appendectomy patient who wants Demerol around the clock for three days postsurgically. Nurses sometimes react to this type of patient by thinking that they might as well give him the medication; it is charted, and he will only tell his doctor if they do not. The light is answered, the medication neatly injected into the upper right maximus gluteus, and the patient is told that we hope he will be feeling better soon. But the intonation of the voice tells the patient how the nurse is really feeling, and the patient will pick up her attitude. The light will probably be on again in three hours. There is a strong chance that what the patient is really feeling is tremendous insecurity.

If the nurse perceived the good patient as someone recuperating at a medically sound rate, she could develop an erroneous attitude toward this type of person. This would be a faulty perception. All patients react to their own realities, and adapt or fail to adapt those realities to the restraints of their environment. One surgical patient may, as illustrated, request pain medication every few hours, while another will resist medication and try to fight through his pain. One patient will be up and walking the halls the day after surgery, and it may take his physician, family, and half the nursing staff to cajole another out of his bed. Neither is a good nor a bad patient. They are merely different. So we have to look at the patient who is recuperating, not only at the medically estimated time but at the patient's estimated time, because the patient does know how he feels and can estimate his own recuperation. Take time to listen to the patient. It could very well be that he does have a low threshold of pain. The nurse could explain that exercise and moving around would decrease the pain because the patient would be using his muscles. A relaxing backrub or some extra attention to the patient's grooming might give him a better self-image and subsequently more confidence to participate in his own recuperation. There was a time in nursing when we thought patient conversation consisted of "Good morning" and "How are you feeling?" In those days, if a patient asked about medication, we replied that we were terribly sorry, we could not tell him, but he would have to take the pill because his doctor wanted him to. We should have grown way beyond this in contemporary nurse–patient communication. Sometimes, when you really talk to a patient, you will discover that he is angry and hostile and that attitude will directly affect how he recuperates and reacts to the set of rules that hospitalization imposes upon him. Communication is necessary, but we must not delude ourselves into thinking that communication is accomplished every time the brain is connected to the mouth, because the resulting words are not always what the patient hears. He hears the intonation of those words, sees the facial expression, and notes the position of the arms. When a nurse goes into a patient's room with a clipboard in front of her or her arms tightly entwined across her chest, she has turned her patient off. The old days when nurses made rounds looking very officious or standoffish are gone, and should be. Naturally, nurses should maintain a professional air. They do not have to be on the patient's level either down or up, but they must approach the patient in a manner that will allow him to express his own realities. If the patient tells how he is really feeling, the nursing goal of a good recovery will be achieved much more rapidly and much more effectively.

In nursing, concepts of good and bad should be restricted to care given and recuperative progress. These conceptual labels should never be applied to the patients themselves. In some nursing situations, the good/bad concept is applied to patient behavior. The bad patient is approached as a problem person, rather than a person with a problem, while the good patient is lavished with tolerance even when he is malingering or when his recovery is going badly. In this unfortunate context, the bad patient is the one who gives the nurse or nursing staff a difficult time. He is recognizable by his behavior, which is hostile and aimed with unerring accuracy at the staff. He rings his bell constantly and complains bitterly when it is not answered within seconds. He is insulting and aggressive with the nurses, ridicules the food and care, or bothers the other patients with imagined wrongs, and he, generally, does one or all of these things at the worst possible time, during the busiest hours of the shift or during a crisis. In many nurses, this kind of behavior elicits an equally negative response. They become punitive and punish the patient in many petty little ways. There is no infraction of safe nursing procedures, usually, but the bad patient's light is answered last, he is left a little longer than necessary on the bed pan, or the spinach he has so often and loudly mentioned hating keeps appearing on his lunch tray. When the nurse speaks to the bad patient, she is polite, clearly enunciating her words while she tells him of her true disapproval in an impressive array of nonverbal behaviors. The patient gets the message.

The good patient is nonthreatening. He does not challenge the nurse's authority or complain as he placidly accepts whatever comes his way. If he is dying, he has the good grace not to upset the nurse by discussing that final reality with her, and when feeling insecure and pushed beyond his limit, he quietly crawls into a fetal position and turns his face to the wall. This patient's bell is answered as promptly as possible, and he is treated to all the little "extras" that the nurse can manage for him. This is wrong, and is in diametric contrast to all that is admirable in nursing and nursing attributes. Nurses dedicate their professional lives to the welfare of the patients committed to their care, and that means all of the patients, not just the ones who are pleasant, nonthreatening, and easy to manage.

In dealing with a patient who presents a problem, the nurse who responds in a punitive manner is playing the patient's game. She is inclined to overlook aspects of the patient's behavior that can be directed toward his recovery. Frequently, an aggressive patient is the best patient in terms of recuperation. He can be helped to direct his energies toward positive recuperative steps. He can actively participate in his own recovery, rather than passively accepting procedures that are done to him and for him. The aggressive patient's energies will not be redirected, however, without effective communication. If he is labeled a bad patient and, in turn, views the nursing staff as indifferent, the potential will never be realized, and his hospitalization will be much less beneficial to him than it should be. The major barrier to recuperation is misunderstanding. The nurse interprets the patient's behavior as directed at her, and the patient reads the nurse's response to the pressures of her own time and priorities as indifference to his needs. Many nurses see time as the basic problem. Too often, they are too busy. In many instances, they feel, their demanding schedules prohibit them from taking the time to talk to patients. This is a valid argument. The increased pressures in professional nursing have tended to limit the patient care time. Leadership demands, paperwork, documentation, staffing, in-service, and other nursing tasks have infringed on patient care time, just as the weight of numbers has effected the allotment of time available for each individual patient. The resulting problem is twofold. First, serious attention should be given to the development of new systems and/or new paraprofessionals to relieve the nurse and allow her more patient time. Secondly, until new approaches can be developed, nurses must be concerned with the quality of the time spent with each patient.

We have touched upon quality of time many times in this text because until nurses can be freed to devote more time to patients, they must be involved in improving the time that is available.

Quality of time can best be improved by communication, especially nonverbal communication. A patient, for example, may be angry because he has been left too long on the bedpan. His calls have not been answered. He does not know that the shift is short on personnel or that there has been an emergency situation a few doors away; he only knows that his distress call has not been answered promptly. He is likely to aim his anger at the nurse who responds to his light, even if it is the first time he has seen that particular nurse. When walking into this situation, we have to remember two things: (1) the patient's anger is not really personal; he is not questioning the competency of the nurse present; nor does he dislike her; he is reacting with anger to an upsetting situation; (2) the patient's anger is justified; he does not know the circumstances that have caused the delay; he experiences his own discomfort and sees the lack of immediate attention to his problem as an indication of disinterest on the part of the nursing staff.

If the nurse reacts to the patient's anger by saying something like: "After all, Mr. Jones, we do have other patients, we are busy. . .," she is investing her limited patient care time poorly. Instead, she should recognize the delay and the fact that it has increased the patient's discomfort by saying: "I'm sorry I couldn't get to you sooner, Mr. Jones, we had an emergency and this is my first opportunity to answer your call." The nurse might take an extra minute or two to make Mr. Jones comfortable and, before leaving, ask if there is anything else she can do for him. Most patients do understand this, and they will respond positively when we give them the opportunity.

THE PATIENTS TALK BACK _____

In compiling this section, we interviewed fifty formerly hospitalized patients. We avoided questions that concerned the caliber of medical care, but focused on their feeling toward their nurses. Those questioned ranged in age from twenty to sixty-two, and were almost equally divided between men and women. The comments varied, but most of those interviewed mentioned one nursing habit that they found particularly irksome. As the nurse first enters the patient's room, after admission, she usually introduces herself by saying "Mary" (or) "John," I'm Miss Smith." This practice seems quite general, and a twenty-two-year-old nurse apparently uses it as readily with a sixty-year-old patient as she does with a twenty-year-old contemporary. Many people see this as a put-down or an attempt to establish dominance. The patient, as we have already discussed, has been temporarily stripped of some of his identity during the admission procedure. He may view the first name/last name introduction as another indignity. Some people even see this type of introduction as the first step of an orientation in which the nurse communicates behavioral expectations to the patient in the same manner as an adult might to a child. They received the message that their hospitalization would be more comfortable if they conformed and did not give anyone a bad time. Many former patients admitted to having been intimidated by the nurses. These people claimed that they were overly solicitous with the nursing staff, because they were afraid their care would be affected if any of the nurses became angry with them. Some patients prefer to be addressed by their first name, but they will generally tell the nurse, and until they do, it is advisable to use the family name. Comments were also made on the use of names in geriatric facilities, where patients are sometimes referred to as "sweetie" or "granny." Most families do not like this any more than most patients do, as expressed by one lady in a geriatric facility who responded to a nurse's "How are we today, granny?" with "I am not your grandmother, so don't call me granny." When we do not know how to address a patient, the simplest solution is simply to ask him what he would like to be called.

A consistent complaint of the former patients was that night nurses seemingly don't care. They take forever to answer the call light. Perhaps patients are a little more critical of night shift personnel than is fair. But we must realize that time and place take on different shades in the hospital. Eleven p.m. may feel like two a.m. to a patient, and to him it seems like an hour waiting for the bell to be answered when, in fact, it may only be a few minutes. But pain at two in the morning is different from pain at two in the afternoon. It takes on another connotation. During the day, the patient feels more secure; he has visitors and there are people walking around. In the middle of the night, he is alone. As a rule, night nurses are less tuned into patient communication than day nurses. They have less opportunity to interact with the patient. The night nurse is frequently task directed because she has to get the charts done, clean the utility cupboard, and go over the doctors orders. When she answers a patient's call, she usually goes on tiptoe into the room with a flashlight turned toward her feet; all the patient sees is the bottom part of her body approaching him. Instead, she should speak softly to the patient, and touch him or his bed so he recognizes her as a care deliverer rather than a white shadow behind a flashlight.

One of the patients in the interview group had more experience with night personnel than the others, and saw them in a very positive light.

> The first night after surgery, I began to hemorrhage. It must have been about midnight. My doctor was called, and he stopped the bleeding. I especially remember the two nurses who were on duty; they helped him, and, after he left, they cleaned me up. I was really a mess, but they were very gentle and kind with me. After a few days, I got to feeling a little better, and I'm a night person, so I was usually awake for a few hours of the night shift. I got to know those two nurses better, and they were really nice. I wasn't well enough to read or anything, so I would just lay there alone in the dark. It was awful, so I asked the nurses if they could leave my door open; they did and I felt so much better just being able to see people move past. One of the two nurses would come in every so often to see if I were awake and needed anything. When they weren't too busy, they would talk to me for a few minutes and I really appreciated that. The night before my discharge, one of them was off. I was so sorry to have missed seeing and thanking her, I wrote her a note. Those two were really good nurses.

Patients also have the concept of good and bad in nursing care, and they perceive good and bad mainly from the nurse's behavior. Only a small percentage of patients have the background or sophistication to judge the quality of a procedure. Therefore, patients who speak of bad nursing care often do not mean that there was no care or that nursing procedures were done incorrectly. They mean they perceived the nurse's behavior toward them as bad—the nurse appeared indifferent, callous, or cold. She looked at the patient with disgust, handled him roughly, ridiculed him, responded to his needs slowly or not at all, or boxed him into a situation that increased his emotional or physical stress. On the patients' rating scale, a good nurse is one who is gentle, kind, and willing to listen to them. Verbally, she shares with the patient, answers his questions, and makes suggestions that will enhance his recuperation. Nonverbally, she handles the patient gently, listens, approaches him nonjudgmentally, and treats him with dignity. Since nursing time is limited, all communication with the patient should be therapeutic and goal directed; the prime goal is always the patient's benefit. Chatter and gossip are not elements of therapeutic communication. One of the interview group was upset by a young staff nurse who kept the patient informed of all the hospital gossip. It disturbed the patient, and she felt it undermined her confidence in the care she was receiving.

Growing Patient Awareness

We all recognize that both nurses and nursing have changed tremendously over the past fifty years. But until we think about it, it may not be quite as apparent that patients have also changed. The past few decades have brought about an awareness of individual rights never before experienced in this country. Ethnic, religious minorities, and women are all aware of their rights, insisting upon fairer treatment and more dignity. This social change reverberates to encompass the nursing situation. Patients are more sensitive to the nursing response. More and more of them are willing to assume the added responsibility that increased freedom implies. A growing number of Americans are interested in staying healthy, as evidenced by the popularity of health food centers, books on staying healthy, and health-oriented exercise. A new kind of health care may be in its infancy, which is called variously: the new medicine, holistic health, or holistic medicine. Practitioners of holistic health include medical doctors, nurses, therapists, psychologists, nutritionists, masseurs, acupuncture specialists, yoga instructors, and many others from both traditional and nontraditional healing arts. One of the focuses of traditional medicine in the 1970s is preventive medicine, since the cost of preventing disease is minor in comparison to the cost of healing it. Both the concept of preventive medicine and holistic health fix some of the responsibility for the state of his health on the individual. If one or either of these concepts gains momentum in the coming years, the nurse will once again see a change in role.

The nurse will become more and more involved in teaching the patient how to preserve his health. An ulcer patient might undergo surgery; his postoperative care would then be designed to include information on what changes in his life style would help prevent another ulcer. The patient will be much more involved in his care than patients are today. He might be present when the staff discusses his care plan, given the effects and side effects of medication, and then given the option of whether or not to take it. If we are moving toward a concept in medicine that will allow the individual more responsibility for his own well-being, nurses should begin now to help their patients assume an active role. This can be accomplished by treating the patient with dignity, allowing him all possible options in his care plan, satisfying his questions with valid answers, and helping him understand his illness and any possible limitations it presents for his future.

YESTERDAY, TODAY, AND TOMORROW

Nurses of the Florence Nightingale era would have difficulty functioning in a modern nursing setting. The technology of our age has left its mark on medicine and nursing. Specialization has been one of the most important factors in nursing during the last few decades. We have the nursing ICU/CCU, geriatric, pediatric, and surgical specialists, to name but a few. To accommodate the technological growth, nursing education has concentrated on procedural techniques and pharmacology. Yet, the procedure learned this year may be replaced by a new one to be learned next year. The nursing profession is not likely to become any more static than it has been in the past decades. New career opportunities for nurses are opening in the areas of hospital management, restorative home health management, and community based nursing. Technology, pharmacology, procedures, environment, and social structure will continue to be fluid, changing from year to year, decade to decade. Yet one element of nursing does not vary. We deal, as nurses, with other human beings. We are involved with the maintenance, restoration, or improvement of their health, and to accomplish our goal we must relate to them on a one-to-one basis. This is an unalterable truth of nursing, and it applies equally to the team nurse and the community based nurse. There can be no nurse–patient relationship without communication. Therapeutic communication will benefit the patient, and it cannot be achieved only by speaking the words we think the patient hears. Therapeutic communication encompasses all of our nonverbal behaviors. It takes time and thought and insight to learn nonverbal communication. It takes more time and effort to become good at it. But once learned, it is ours. We will not have to relearn it next year. Whatever direction our own career follows, nonverbal communication will enable us to reach more of our patients, better express our intent, deliver better care and more patient benefits, and make nursing a more personally rewarding experience.

Bibliography Notes

1. Kron, Thora. *Communication in Nursing.* 2nd Ed., Philadelphia: W. B. Saunders, 1967, p. 40.
2. Dance, F. E. X. *Toward a Theory of Human Communication.* New York: Holt, Rinehart, & Winston, 1967, p. 290.
3. Orlando, Ida Jean. *The Dynamic Nurse–Patient Relationship.* New York: G. P. Putnam's Sons, 1961.
4. Roberts, Sharon. *Behavioral Concepts and the Critically Ill Patient.* Englewood Cliffs, New Jersey: Prentice-Hall, 1976, p. 274.
5. Darwin, Charles. *The Expression of the Emotions in Man and Animals.* London: John Murray, 1872.
6. Ekman, Paul, and Wallace V. Friesen. *Unmasking the Face.* Englewood Cliffs, New Jersey: Prentice-Hall, 1975.
7. Skipper, James, and Robert C. Leonard. *Social Interaction and Patient Care.* Philadelphia: J. B. Lippincott, 1965.
8. Barbara, Dominick A. *The Art of Listening.* Springfield, Illinois: Charles C Thomas, 1966.
9. Barnlund, Dean C. *Interpersonal Communication—Survey and Studies.* 2nd Ed., New York: W. W. Norton, & Co., 1963.
10. Erikson, Erik. *Childhood and Society.* 2nd Ed., New York: W. W. Norton, 1963.

11. Le Boyer, Frederick. *Birth without Violence.* New York: Alfred A. Knopf, 1976, pp. 59–60.
12. Davitz, Lois Jean. *Interperson Process in Nursing: Case Histories.* New York: Springer, 1970.
13. *R.N. Magazine,* Comprehension Chart. New Jersey: Medical Economics, February 1976.
14. Lieberman, Morton A. "Psychological Correlates of Impending Death: Some Preliminary Observations." *Journal of Gerontology,* Vol. 20, No. 2, pp. 181–190, February 1965.
15. Kübler-Ross, Elisabeth. *On Death and Dying.* New York: Macmillan, 1969, pp. 419–430.
16. Frankl, Viktor E. *Man's Search for Meaning: An Introduction to Logo Therapy.* New York: Washington Square Press, 1969, pp. 27, 121, 125.
17. Engel, George L. *Psychological Development in Health and Disease.* Philadelphia, W. B. Saunders, 1964, p. 85.

Bibliography

Barbara, Dominick A. *The Art of Listening.* Springfield, Illinois: Charles C Thomas, 1966.

Barnlund, Dean C. *Interpersonal Communication—Survey and Studies.* New York: Houghton Mifflin, 1968.

Birdwhistell, R. "Kinesics and Communication," in E. Carpenter and M. McLuhan (eds.). *Explorations in Communication.* New York: Beacon, 1960.

Dance, F. E. X. "Toward a Theory of Human Communication." in F. E. X. Dance (ed.). *Human Communication Theory.* New York: Holt, Rinehart & Winston, 1967.

Darwin, Charles. *The Expression of the Emotions in Man and Animals.* London: John Murray, 1872. (current edition: University of Chicago Press, 1965).

Davitz, Lois Jean. "Nonverbal Vocal Communication of Feeling," *The Journal of Communication,* Vol. 11, No. 1, pp. 81–86, June 1961.

Ekman, Paul, and Wallace V. Friesen. *Unmasking the Face.* Englewood Cliffs, New Jersey: Prentice-Hall, 1975.

Engel, George L. *Psychological Development in Health and Disease.* Philadelphia: W. B. Saunders, 1964.

Erikson, Erik. *Childhood and Society.* 2nd Ed., New York: W. W. Norton, 1963.

Frankl, Viktor E. *Man's Search for Meaning: An Introduction to Logotherapy.* New York: Washington Square Press, 1969.

Illich, Ivan. *The Medical Nemesis.* New York: Pantheon, 1976.

Kimmel, Douglas C. *Adulthood and Aging.* New York: John Wiley & Sons, 1974.

Kron, Thora. *Communication in Nursing.* 2nd Ed., Philadelphia: W. B. Saunders, 1972.

Kübler-Ross, Elisabeth. *On Death and Dying.* New York: Macmillan, 1969.

Le Boyer, Frederick. *Birth Without Violence.* New York: Alfred A. Knopf, 1976.

Lieberman, Morton A. "Psychological Correlates of Impending Death: Some Preliminary Observations," *The Journal of Gerontology,* Vol. 20, No. 2, pp. 181–190, February 1965.

Orlando, Ida Jean. *The Dynamic Nurse-Patient Relationship.* New York: G. P. Putnam's Sons, 1961.

R.N. Magazine. "Comprehension Chart." Oradell, New Jersey: Medical Economics, February 1976.

Roberts, Sharon. *Behavioral Concepts and the Critically Ill Patient.* Englewood Cliffs, New Jersey: Prentice-Hall, 1976.

Skipper, James, and Robert C. Leonard. *Social Interaction and Patient Care.* Philadelphia: J. B. Lippincott, 1965.

Recommended Reading

Allport, Gordon W. *Becoming*. New Haven: Yale University Press, 1955.

Axline, Virginia. *Dibs in Search of Self*. New York: Ballantine Books, 1964.

Brown, Martha Montgomery, and Grace R. Fowler. *Psychodynamic Nursing: A Biosocial Orientation*. Philadelphia; W. B. Saunders, 1971.

Davitz, Joel R., et al. *The Communication of Emotional Meaning*. New York: McGraw-Hill, 1964.

Dewey, John, and Arthur F. Bently. *Knowing and the Known*. Boston: Beacon, 1949.

Frankl, Viktor E. *Man's Search for Meaning*. New York: Washington Square Press, 1969.

Fromm, Erich. *The Art of Loving*. New York: Harper & Row, Bantam, 1956.

Fromm, Erich. *The Forgotten Language*. New York: Rinehart, 1951.

Hall, Edward T. *The Silent Language*. Connecticut: Fawcett, 1959.

Kalkman, Marion, and Anne Davis. *New Dimensions in Mental Health Psychiatric Nursing*. New York, McGraw-Hill, 1974.

Katz, Robert L. *Empathy: Its Nature and Uses*. New York: Free Press of Glencoe, 1963.

Keyes, Joan, and Charles Hofling. *Basic Psychiatric Concepts in Nursing*. Philadelphia: Lippincott, 1974.

Kron, Thora. *Communication in Nursing*. Philadelphia: W. B. Saunders, 1967.

Lockerby, Florence. *Communication for Nurses*. St. Louis: C. V. Mosby, 1958.

Marcel, Gabriel. *Being and Having: An Existentialist Diary.* New York: Harper & Row, 1965.

Maslow, A. H. *The Farther Reaches of Human Nature.* New York: Viking Press, 1971.

Matson, Floyd, and Ashley Montague. (eds.) *The Human Dialogue, Perspectives on Communication.* New York: Free Press, 1967.

May, Rollo (ed.). *Existence: A New Dimension in Psychiatry and Psychology.* New York: Random House, 1960.

Orlando, Ida Jean. *The Dynamic Nurse-Patient Relationship.* New York: G. P. Putnam's Sons, 1961.

Patterson, Josephine G., and Loretta T. Zderad. *Humanistic Nursing.* New York: John Wiley & Sons, 1976.

Peplau, Hildegard. *Interpersonal Relations in Nursing.* New York: G. P. Putnam's Sons, 1952.

Rogers, Carl R., and Barry Stevens. *Person to Person: The Problem of Being Human.* Lafayette, California: Real People Press, 1967.

Ruesch, Jurgen. *Therapeutic Communication.* New York: W. W. Norton, 1961.

Ruesch, Jurgen, and Weldon Kees. *Nonverbal Communication.* Berkeley: University of California Press, 1956.

Skipper, James, and Robert C. Leonard. *Social Interaction and Patient Care.* Philadelphia: J. B. Lippincott, 1965.

Stevens, Barry. *Don't Push the River.* Lafayette, California: Real People Press, 1970.

Tillich, Paul. *The Courage to Be.* New Haven: Yale University Press, 1952.

Travelbee, Joyce. *Interpersonal Aspects of Nursing.* Philadelphia: F. A. Davis, 1966.

Index